"What this book says is an eye-opener. I am one of those people who no longer have a social life because of IBS. This book has made a difference for me. How very kind of you to write this for those of us who need it so desperately!"

—*Barbara Andersen, IBS sufferer*

"Thank you for this information. It has helped me far more than any doctor has. I have been using this guide for some time now, and I am like a new person, back to feeling like me. Your suggestions have become mainstays in my eating habits."

—*Pat Schultz, IBS sufferer*

"Thank you, thank you, thank you! This information is so wonderful and complete that I can't believe it hasn't been taught as a requirement in medical school. I read it and read it again, and carry it with me when I travel. I feel so hopeful. I have been following the eating guidelines and I feel like a new person. I can't believe it! No cramping, no explosive liquid 'you know what.' When I first got this diet recommendation I thought yeah, right, like this is gonna help. But I had nothing to lose except the misery and Wow! what a difference this diet has made. Following this diet has been the biggest help in dealing with my IBS. I recommend it to everyone."

—*Diane Feierabend, IBS sufferer*

"I cannot tell you how valuable this information is for someone who has suffered with IBS all his life."

—*Steven Segal, IBS sufferer*

"I am 100 percent better. Your advice and diet information opened my eyes to a whole new way of eating. I thank you for sharing your information with me. People need to know about IBS—I know many suffer in silence. Maybe if more people knew about it and how to help, it wouldn't be such a curse. Just reading this information over made me feel better. It's like you wrote everything especially for me—this is how much I identified with everything you said. Thanks a bunch. I really appreciate this information."

—*Crystal Boggs, IBS sufferer*

"I can't seem to say enough about your diet. I have been raving to anyone who will listen. Your cookbook is fabulous, with great recipes and nutrition information."

—*Jill Sklar, Crohn's sufferer*

EATING FOR
I·B·S

175 DELICIOUS, NUTRITIOUS,

LOW-FAT, LOW-RESIDUE

RECIPES TO STABILIZE

THE TOUCHIEST TUMMY

HEATHER VAN VOROUS

Da Capo
LIFE
LONG

A MEMBER OF THE PERSEUS BOOKS GROUP

Cataloging-in-Publication data for this book is available from the Library of Congress.

ISBN: 978-1-56924-600-9

Published by Da Capo Press
A Member of the Perseus Books Group
www.dacapopress.com

Note: The information in this book is true and complete to the best of our knowledge. This book is intended only as an informative guide for those wishing to know more about health issues. In no way is this book intended to replace, countermand, or conflict with the advice given to you by your own physician. The ultimate decision concerning care should be made between you and your doctor. We strongly recommend you follow his or her advice. Information in this book is general and is offered with no guarantees on the part of the authors or Da Capo Press. The authors and publisher disclaim all liability in connection with the use of this book. The names and identifying details of people associated with events described in this book have been changed. Any similarity to actual persons is coincidental.

Da Capo Press books are available at special discounts for bulk purchases in the U.S. by corporations, institutions, and other organizations. For more information, please contact the Special Markets Department at the Perseus Books Group, 2300 Chestnut Street, Suite 200, Philadelphia, PA, 19103, or call (800) 255-1514, or e-mail special.markets@perseusbooks.com.

30 29 28

With all my love to Grams and Bumpa . . .

and all my heart to Will.

CONTENTS

∞

AUTHOR'S NOTE

∞

I LEARNED HOW TO cook from my beloved grandmother, Marion Wille Orcutt, who is now stricken with Alzheimer's and tenderly cared for by my grandfather, Donald Orcutt. As a gift in their names, a percentage of all author's proceeds from this book will go directly to the Alzheimer's Association of America.

ACKNOWLEDGMENTS

∞

ANY VERY TALENTED and kind people helped me with this book, and I would like them to know how much I appreciate their time and effort. Thank you to Matthew Lore, an editor far better than I had even dared hope for, and a very nice guy as well. Thanks also to Susi Oberhelman, for a lovely cover design; Pauline Neuwirth, for her terrific interior design; and Ghadah Alrawi and Sue McCloskey for all their help. Thank you to Ling Lucas and Janis Donnaud, wonderful agents who took a chance on someone new. Thank you to Jill Sklar and Bella Nissen, for always being there, and for sharing such great information, provocative questions, and unfailing good humor. Thank you to Shawn Eric Case and Jeffrey Roberts, for their kindness and encouragement, unrelenting support of all IBS sufferers, and heroic efforts to publicize IBS. To Meg Wilson and DeLynne Higginbotham, my partners-in-crime, thanks for laughs and boundless enthusiasm. For Mom, who believed in me from day one and never doubted this book for a moment. To everyone on the internet IBS boards and all of the wonderful people who E-mailed me for help—you know who you are. And for Will, who deserves a co-author credit, because without him this book would never have been written. Thank you.

INTRODUCTION

∞

$\mathcal{A}$LTHOUGH AN ESTIMATED 15 to 20 percent of all Americans, or 39 to 52 million people, have Irritable Bowel Syndrome (IBS), there is slight media attention given to the subject and precious little medical research conducted. IBS is an incurable condition; there is no alternative to controlling the symptoms through daily diet. Yet incredibly, many doctors, dieticians, and nutritionists appear to be either wholly uninformed or wildly misinformed about the eating requirements for IBS. I don't know why this is, but I do know things must change. I hope this book will help.

Until I wrote *Eating for IBS* I had never met another person with Irritable Bowel Syndrome. I have yet to meet someone without IBS who truly appreciates how devastating and excruciating the condition can be. It is literally ruining people's lives—there are many folks out there with IBS who are afraid to leave their homes, who cannot work, drive, socialize, or travel. They live each day in fear. The illness has an unimaginably dramatic effect on every single aspect of their lives, and yet, they often cannot even get their own family, friends, employers, and doctors to acknowledge that they have a legitimate physical problem. They feel that they are treated like hypochondriacs, and that their complaints are either summarily dismissed or met with outright contempt.

I know firsthand the sheer brutality of pain that characterizes an IBS attack (imagine someone setting their hand on fire, then plunging it into your lower abdomen to try to rip your guts out), so I empathize unconditionally with all of these people. I know exactly what they are going through because I have been there myself. The only reason I am able to lead a normal life is because I follow the dietary advice in this book.

I have had IBS since I was nine years old, although I went undiagnosed for six long years. My pediatrician at the time refused to send me for diagnostic tests because my symptoms didn't fit any disorder she knew (though I was a textbook case), and therefore the problem was all in my head. This doctor also dismissed my suffering as "only pain." She flatly told me that my symptoms did not warrant treatment and that I should "quit whining." I was in the fourth grade at the time and had recently fainted from pain in a neighbor's garden.

When I was eventually diagnosed (by a different doctor) at the age of fifteen, I was offered little help beyond being given the label "IBS." Although it was a relief to finally have a name for my problem, I was not provided with any dietary advice whatsoever. My doctor simply prescribed an anti-spasmodic drug and recommended Metamucil. It took a great many years of daily trial and error, and excruciatingly painful experience, to gradually learn which foods triggered my IBS and which soothed it. It required additional medical research to realize precisely why these foods had the physical effects they did, be they hurtful or helpful.

However, even after learning exactly what I could and couldn't eat as well as the reasons why, it was still very difficult at times to follow the IBS diet. Most typical American meals, whether home-cooked or in restaurants, were simply intolerable. What I needed was a way to bridge the gap between knowing *what* to eat and *how*. I wasn't about to sacrifice my health, nor was I willing to forego great food, so I had to find a way to create recipes that were both safe (and I use the word "safe" deliberately, knowing how justifiably fearful many IBS sufferers are when it comes to food) *and* scrumptious. The happy result was that by following the IBS diet I was led unexpectedly to a life of culinary adventure, and along the way I developed a cooking strategy that's surprisingly simple, fun, and delicious.

How did this happen? Well, instead of viewing IBS food guidelines as a dietary prison sentence to be borne with grim determination, I took them as an opportunity to explore new cuisines, as an incentive to take control of my own health and life, and as an invitation to practice a little kitchen wizardry. This often meant exploring techniques from different culinary traditions and cultures. One important lesson I learned early on was that delicious American homestyle cooking was amazingly easy to adapt to the IBS kitchen—the key was simply clever substitutions, *never* deprivation. A second realization was that ethnic cooking frequently offered the most exciting variety of foods as well as some of the most easily modified recipes. Finally, I learned that even if a recipe adaptation failed miserably, the dog would always eat it.

Once I had decided to view IBS dietary restrictions as mere challenges to be met through creative thinking and cooking, I realized that I had a whole world of cuisines to explore, exotic foods to taste, and nothing at all to lose by trying different things. I vowed to never be intimidated by new cooking techniques, specialty ingredients, or recipes from different traditions and cultures. Food is fun, cooking is a pleasure, and eating a delicious meal is the wonderful end reward. After I had gained the knowledge that allowed me to eat without fear, I refused to be afraid in the kitchen. Recipes just couldn't be too varied, exciting, or interesting—safe *never* meant boring or bland. And like everything else that seems daunting at first, with practice came comfort, and with repetition came familiarity. New techniques were never as complicated as they had initially seemed once I actually tried them, and ethnic foods were no longer foreign once I had tasted them. Recipe adaptations soon became a quick and easy matter, and it grew quite clear that there was simply no limit to great taste when it came to cooking for IBS.

My personal IBS recipe collection accumulated gradually over the years, eventually filling an entire shelf of notebooks in my kitchen bookcase with a wide variety of exciting, delicious, and healthy dishes. As I was the only person I knew with IBS, however, these recipes, as well as the dietary guidelines that formed them, were simply for my own use. It never occurred to me—in fact, it didn't seem possible—that there were other people (millions of them!) suffering from the same problem I had, who could all be helped by my information. Then the internet came along and changed everything. How, exactly? Well, *Eating for IBS* evolved over the course of a few years from an E-mail file I created to send to other people on IBS boards.

I had surfed onto these web sites with a casual interest at first, because I don't give too much thought to my own IBS anymore. I've lived with it on a daily basis for so long that I automatically control my diet, and thus the symptoms, through habit. So I was completely astonished and appalled by how much the people on the IBS boards were suffering, and by the fact that no one had told them how to eat properly. Many of their stories were heartbreaking, and their desperation was palpable. They felt they were treated with a complete lack of respect by doctors and offered no help at all—many were told things like "stop complaining," and "the pain can't be as bad as you say or you'd kill yourself." These were people whose lives were so utterly compromised by IBS that they attempted suicide, purchased RVs with toilets in the back so they could drive without worrying about a sudden attack, and wore adult diapers every day in case they were stricken in public and couldn't make it to a restroom in time.

I was deeply affected by the stories on the IBS boards, so I started compiling all the advice I had to give, and eventually this information turned into a full-fledged eating plan. I added the recipes when I realized that most people would be dumbstruck when told they could no longer eat meat, dairy, fried foods, coffee, or soda pop. I didn't want people to feel that there was nothing left they could eat, and I knew that's how most of them would react to my information. There is in fact a wealth of wonderful things to eat that don't trigger IBS attacks, and as I had created hundreds of dishes over the years, I decided to share my recipes along with the dietary advice.

I then did some research to verify and annotate the accuracy of my medical/nutritional information (documented through extensive footnotes in the text so that readers may consult more technical and detailed authorities at the primary source). I also read a copy of every IBS book on the market. I have to admit I had a very hard time believing that there was nothing with accurate dietary information already out there, despite what I heard from the people on the IBS boards. It was shocking to discover they were absolutely right—the books available had dietary advice that ranged from worthless to downright dangerous. One book's outrageous suggestions made me so angry I nearly threw it across the room. Had the author been standing there I think I would have smacked him, as he clearly had no comprehension of the physical torment people with IBS endure, let alone any sympathy for their suffering. I turned my E-mail file into a full-fledged book after learning that there really was no legitimate IBS dietary information, and certainly no comprehensive eating guide with recipes, anywhere on the market.

I was helped immensely along the way by the terrific comments I received from fellow IBS sufferers via E-mail. Their feedback was invaluable. The questions they asked had a very humbling effect, as I came to realize just how seriously people were taking the advice that I sent them. Here I was a total stranger, an anonymous nobody sending them E-mail, and they were following every recommendation I had given them to the letter. This really drove home the fact that they had no other source of information—virtually all that they knew about how to control their IBS through diet they had learned from me and my E-mail file. These people really provided the inspiration to see this project through, and the determination to get the information into the hands of everyone who needs it.

The end result was this, the first and only book about Irritable Bowel Syndrome written by someone who personally has IBS and has learned to effectively control the problem through diet. I honestly believe that this is also the first and only book to offer IBS sufferers the information they need to live a normal life by explicitly detailing how to manage IBS through eating habits. My conviction in this matter is backed not only by decades of firsthand experience but by the feedback from hundreds of other IBS sufferers. IBS is not a mental problem, nor is it strictly stress-induced, nor can it be solved through drugs or surgery. It is a problem that must be addressed on a daily basis through diet. The general guidelines and explicit recommendations in this book have helped everyone with IBS who has followed the advice. It is safe to assume that the information can in some way assist all IBS sufferers—the syndrome is not so highly individualized that no dietary generalizations can be made, because the colon reacts to specific foods in predictable ways. This is basic biology.

What I hope will be one of this book's major revelations is that, contrary to what people may think, eating for IBS does not mean deprivation, never going to restaurants, eating boring or bland food, or an unhealthily limited diet. There are safe recipes for traditional homestyle cooking, ethnic foods, rich desserts, snacks, and party foods. There is never any need to sacrifice an ounce of flavor or visual flair to create a gourmet IBS meal. As a result, it's quite easy to cook for others following IBS guidelines without people even realizing that the food they're eating is tailored for medical needs. In addition, the IBS diet is inherently healthy (low fat, plant-based), lowers the risk of heart disease and cancer, is slimming, and it's delicious, too. It's easily suitable for an entire family to follow. IBS sufferers do not have to cook weird or special meals for themselves while their families follow a "normal" diet.

In short, people with IBS who follow the advice in this book can achieve their dearest goal: after endless pain and suffering, they can finally eat without fear. I know this to be true because I am one of those people.

EATING FOR
I·B·S

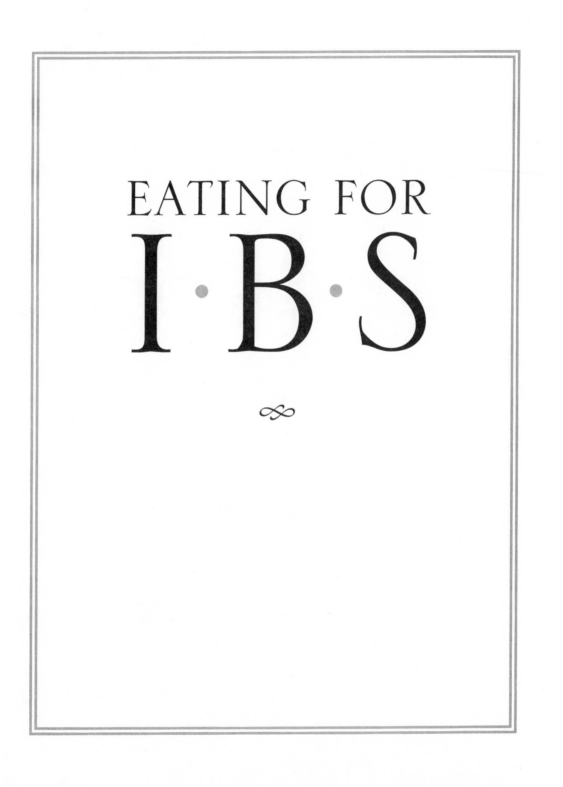

SO WHAT IS IBS, AND HOW DO I KNOW IF I HAVE IT?

∞

*I*BS IS NOT an explicitly defined medical diagnosis with a clearly understood cause. It is actually the term coined by the medical establishment to mean "I don't know what's wrong with you. There are no physical findings that point to a recognizable problem I can treat and cure." Doctors will freely admit this and typically suggest their patients try a combination of dietary changes, stress management techniques,[1] and prescription anti-spasmodic (anti-cholinergic) drugs.[2] There is also a new class of drug, serotonin-antagonists, that shows promise in controlling IBS symptoms.[3]

---

[1] Several stress-reduction treatments have been studied in patients with IBS, including cognitive-behavioral treatment, hypnosis, relaxation, and biofeedback. They appear to be effective in reducing abdominal pain and diarrhea but not constipation. It is not known whether improvement in IBS symptoms relates to changes in gastrointestinal physiology or in the psychological interpretation of enteroceptive sensation. A positive response is associated primarily with patients who relate symptom exacerbations to stressors, and have a waxing and waning of symptoms rather than chronic pain. There is no comparative data to determine which treatment is superior. (*Guidelines of the American Gastroenterological Association.*)

[2] Levsin, Bentyl, Donnatol, Pro-Banthine, Librax, Modulon, Sinequan.

[3] Lotronex, by Glaxo Wellcome, is the first of this new generation of agents being studied specifically for the treatment of multiple symptoms of IBS. The drug works as a potent and selective 5-HT3 antagonist. The neurotransmitter serotonin and 5-HT3 receptors that are extensively distributed in the human gastrointestinal tract are thought to play a role in increasing the sensation of pain and affecting bowel function in patients with IBS. While the precise mechanism of action of Lotronex is not yet fully understood, one hypothesis is that Lotronex blocks the action of serotonin at 5-HT3 receptor sites in the enteric nervous system. Lotronex works best in women and in patients who have diarrhea as their primary symptom.

IBS is a chronic, functional disorder of the gastrointestinal (GI) tract characterized by recurrent abdominal pain and discomfort accompanied by alterations in bowel function, diarrhea, constipation, or a combination of both, typically over months or years. It is not caused by structural, biochemical, or infectious abnormalities, but is instead classified as a "dysregulation" of brain-bowel inter-function. It is worth noting that the gut actually has its own "brain," the enteric nervous system (ENS), which is the only part of the peripheral nervous system that is capable of mediating reflex behavior in the absence of input from the brain or spinal cord. In other words, there is a brain in your bowel that acts completely independent from the brain in your head.[4]

Although there is clearly still much research to be done on IBS, the most recent findings suggest that IBS sufferers have, in sum, colons that are too easily stimulated. IBS has been called an "altered regulation of bowel motor and sensory function; a disturbance in the interaction between the gut, the brain, and the autonomic nervous system which regulates involuntary reactions of internal organs."[5] In other words, people with IBS have colons that react to stimuli that do not affect normal colons, and their reactions are far more severe. The result is heightened pain sensitivity and abnormal gut motility (irregular or increased GI muscle contractions).

This overreaction and hypersensitivity cause the standard symptoms of IBS: lower abdominal pain (frequently severe, and can be to the point of losing consciousness),[6] extreme cramping, vomiting in association with the pain, diarrhea (often sudden and explosive), gas, and bloating. Constipation may follow an attack as the colon "shuts down" in response to the earlier spasms, and can then become an ongoing problem in its own right.

An estimated 15 to 20 percent of all Americans suffer from IBS, more than have asthma or diabetes, and a 60 to 70 percent majority of these people are women.[7] In fact, IBS is the single most common gastrointestinal diagnosis among gastroenterology practices in the US, and it is one of the top ten most frequently diagnosed conditions among all US physicians.[8] The average age of IBS onset is late teens to early twenties, but people can be afflicted in childhood. There is no known "cure," as this problem is a syndrome, not a disease. As such, if you can control the symptoms, you effectively eliminate the problem. I have found that diet alone can alleviate more than 90 percent of the misery of IBS.

[4] See *The Second Brain: A Groundbreaking New Understanding of Nervous Disorders of the Stomach and Intestine*, by Dr. Michael Gershon.
[5] *Participate*, Quarterly Bulletin of the IFFGD, Vol 8, No. 3, Fall 1999, p. 7.
[6] Nearly 40 percent of women with IBS report experiencing abdominal pain they describe as "intolerable." (Citation from the largest, most comprehensive national survey ever conducted on IBS, July/August 1999, by Schulman, Ronca and Bucuvalas, Inc., funded by Glaxo Wellcome.)
[7] International Foundation for Functional Gastrointestinal Disorders.

My favorite analogy is that having IBS is rather like having very sensitive skin, only the problem is internal. You cannot visit a dermatologist to cure sensitive skin, because there is nothing physically wrong that can be fixed. No surgery or drug can eliminate the problem. It is simply a condition that must be controlled on a daily basis by avoiding those things that trigger the symptoms. IBS requires the same type of precautions.

Please note that a diagnosis of IBS is acceptable *only* if the patient has the hallmark symptoms in combination with a lack of physical abnormalities as determined by diagnostic tests. Although published diagnostic guidelines do exist for IBS, almost 80 percent of US physicians say they don't follow them, and less than 20 percent say they are even somewhat familiar with these guidelines.[9]

Food allergies, gluten intolerance disorders such as celiac sprue,[10] inflammatory bowel diseases such as Crohn's and Ulcerative Colitis,[11] colon cancer, endometriosis, and even ovarian cancer can all mimic the symptoms of IBS and must be conclusively ruled out. Removal of the gallbladder or ileum (the last portion of the small intestine) can also result in chronic diarrhea that may be misdiagnosed as IBS. This diarrhea results from the malabsorption of bile acids secreted by the liver—these acids irritate the colon and cause severe diarrhea. The prescription drug Questran, which binds the bile acids in the intestines and prevents them from reaching the colon, can help this problem. On a related note, gallstones can cause daily indigestion, nausea, and bloating, which may also be misdiagnosed as IBS.

If your GI symptoms do not match those of IBS but you are given this diagnosis anyway simply because your doctor cannot find anything structurally wrong with you, *find a new doctor*. It is unacceptable for all patients with unexplainable abdominal symptoms

---

[8] American Gastroenterological Association.

[9] Although 58 percent of US physicians think IBS is easy to diagnose, women with IBS see an average of three physicians over a three-year period before they receive a clear-cut diagnosis. (Citation from the largest, most comprehensive national survey ever conducted on IBS, July/August 1999, by Schulman, Ronca and Bucuvalas, Inc., funded by Glaxo Wellcome.)

[10] Celiac sprue is a genetic, autoimmune disorder that damages the small intestine. People with celiac sprue cannot tolerate gluten, a protein found in wheat, rye, barley, and possibly oats. A simple blood test that measures the levels of gluten-antibodies can diagnose celiac sprue, and the diagnosis can be confirmed with an intestinal biopsy that checks for tissue damage. In the United States, the average time between the onset of celiac sprue symptoms and diagnosis is ten years. The only treatment for this disorder is a gluten-free diet.

[11] It is crucial that a person with an inflammatory bowel disease not be misdiagnosed with IBS, particularly since many doctors offer no help to their IBS patients beyond urging them to "eat more fiber." Should a person with Crohn's or Ulcerative Colitis follow this advice, a sudden increase in their ingestion of insoluble fiber can result in bowel obstructions requiring hospitalization and surgery.

to be lumped into the IBS category and summarily dismissed, but unfortunately this is a common occurrence.[12]

Although the most significant and easily addressed cause of IBS is diet, stress also commonly triggers or exacerbates attacks. Stress inhibits the sympathetic nerve plexuses, while stimulating excessive adrenaline production, which upsets the rhythmic muscle contractions of the GI tract. It is important to note that there are definite variations among individuals in this regard, and that there appear to be two categories of sufferers in terms of colon sensitivity: those whose attacks are triggered solely from stress, who need only control their diets during times of duress to keep symptoms at bay; and those whose attacks are triggered by a combination of foods and stress both, and who must carefully monitor their diets at all times. Additionally, many women find that menstrual cramps will cause IBS to flare, as the excess prostagladins associated with uterine contractions can trigger gastrointestinal spasms. Interestingly, hot and humid weather can also play a role in IBS attacks, in two ways: (1) heat is a stressor, and (2) air pressure changes from humid weather fronts can affect the levels of serotonin in the body, which in turn reduces a person's pain tolerance. Finally, a night without adequate sleep is often directly correlated to IBS attacks the next day.

There is no evidence whatsoever that IBS sufferers fit a typical psychological profile, such as having abusive childhoods or being prone to depression. To the contrary, all reliable research suggests that this is strictly a physical problem and should be treated as such.[13] IBS has not been shown to lead to any other syndrome or disease. No link has been established between IBS and inflammatory bowel diseases such as Crohn's or Ulcerative Colitis. IBS does not lead to colon cancer.[14]

---

[12] Diagnosis of IBS requires a physical examination and the following studies: complete blood count; sedimentation rate; chemistries; stool for ova, parasites, and blood; colonoscopy if older than fifty years; gynecological exam including CA-125 blood test for ovarian cancer. Other diagnostic studies should be minimal and will depend on the symptom subtype. For example, in patients with diarrhea-predominant symptoms, a small bowel radiograph to rule out Crohn's disease, or lactose/dextrose H2 breath test. For patients with pain as the predominant symptom, a plain abdominal radiograph during an acute episode to exclude bowel obstruction and other abdominal pathology. For patients with indigestion, nausea, and bloating, an abdominal ultrasound to rule out gallstones. (Guidelines of the American Gastroenterological Association.)

[13] "IBS is a real, chronic medical condition with painful and potentially debilitating symptoms," says Lin Chang, MD, co-director of the Neuroenteric Disease Program at the University of California at Los Angles Medical School. "Research suggests that IBS stems from a physiologic abnormality, and is clearly not a psychosomatic disorder." (Citation from the largest, most comprehensive national survey ever conducted on IBS, July/August 1999, by Schulman, Ronca and Bucuvalas, Inc., funded by Glaxo Wellcome.)

[14] IBS Information from the National Digestive Diseases Information Clearinghouse (NDDIC). The NDDIC is a service of the National Institute of Diabetes and Digestive and Kidney Diseases, part of the National Institutes of Health, under the US Public Health Service. The clearinghouse, authorized by Congress in 1980, provides information about digestive diseases and health to people with digestive diseases and their families, health care professionals, and the public. The NDDIC answers inquiries; develops, reviews, and distributes publications; and works closely with professional and patient organizations and government agencies to coordinate resources about digestive diseases.

Because so much remains unknown about IBS, there is frequently a great deal of confusion and misunderstanding about the syndrome among patients and physicians alike.[15] This lack of understanding can lead to misdiagnosis and even unnecessary surgery. In particular, women with IBS face an increased risk of unwarranted hysterectomy or ovarian surgery,[16] and their reported rate of abdominal or intestinal surgery (aside from Caesarean sections) is almost double that of women without IBS.[17]

Despite the enormous social and economic costs of IBS (it is the second leading cause of worker absenteeism, behind the common cold),[18] medical research in this area is severely underfunded. IBS receives less than 1 percent of digestive disease research funding through the National Institutes of Health (NIH).[19]

This book is the end result of my personal experience and research, and came about when I realized that every other IBS sufferer I was coming in contact with was desperate for help, as they had been treated as dismissively by their doctors as I was by mine. I have met people whose doctors have told them they are being "silly" because they are unable to leave their house and go to work due to blinding pain and diarrhea. I have met people who have been told that their abdominal pain is "normal," and that suffering from diarrhea up to fourteen times a day is no cause for concern. I have met people whose doctors have told them to "stop whining," or that they "didn't want to hear any more complaining." I have met people who are unable to drive, work, sleep, eat, socialize, and take vacations; in short, unable to live a normal life because they must endure extreme agony every day. Some have even had gastroenterologists tell them that "diet doesn't affect IBS." This is like saying that the air you breathe doesn't affect your lungs.[20]

---

[15] Eighty seven percent of US doctors admit that physicians need better education about IBS. (Citation from the largest, most comprehensive national survey ever conducted on IBS, July/August 1999, by Schulman, Ronca and Bucuvalas, Inc., funded by Glaxo Wellcome.)

[16] International Foundation for Functional Gastrointestinal Disorders.

[17] Citation from the largest, most comprehensive national survey ever conducted on IBS, July/August 1999, by Schulman, Ronca and Bucuvalas, Inc., funded by Glaxo Wellcome.

[18] Women with active IBS take three times as many sick days as women in the general public, miss work or school twice as often, and almost one in four are forced to allow extra time for their daily commute due to abdominal symptoms. (Citation from the largest, most comprehensive national survey ever conducted on IBS, July/August 1999, by Schulman, Ronca and Bucuvalas, Inc., funded by Glaxo Wellcome.)

[19] International Foundation for Functional Gastrointestinal Disorders.

[20] On average, doctors who treat IBS rate the pain felt by their IBS patients as being significantly less severe than the patients themselves report. Furthermore, a majority of doctors say that while IBS may be distressing, it is not a serious medical condition, despite the fact that three out of ten women with IBS report having been hospitalized for their abdominal symptoms at some point. More than one in four women with IBS say that their doctor does not understand how much pain or discomfort they feel and that there is no point in consulting their doctor about their symptoms. Nearly a third of all US physicians mistakenly believe that IBS is primarily a psychological problem. (Citations from the largest, most comprehensive national survey ever conducted on IBS, July/August 1999, by Schulman, Ronca and Bucuvalas, Inc., funded by Glaxo Wellcome.)

I find it inexcusable that so many people are offered no dietary help whatsoever from the medical authorities they consult when it is virtually impossible to control IBS without proper eating habits. The nutritional advice offered in this book should be common knowledge to gastroenterologists, family doctors, nutritionists, and dieticians, and it should be routinely provided to IBS patients. Unfortunately, it is not. As a result, many people continue to suffer needlessly from this syndrome. My hope is that this book will provide people with the information that has dramatically helped me, so that it may in turn help them.

A NEW WAY TO EAT

∞

THE FUNDAMENTAL IDEA of eating for IBS is to avoid foods that over-stimulate the colon, and eat foods that soothe and regulate it. This is best accomplished by strictly limiting the amount of dietary **fat** (the single most powerful digestive tract stimulant); eating **soluble** fiber (low-residue foods) consistently with every snack and meal; eliminating coffee, carbonated beverages, and alcohol; being very careful with **insoluble** fiber (high-residue foods); and avoiding overeating by having frequent small meals instead of large ones. It is also important to avoid cigarettes, because tobacco wreaks havoc on the digestive tract.

FRINGE BENEFITS!

The IBS diet follows the FDA Food Pyramids. Eating safely for IBS will lower your risk of heart disease, cancer, arthritis, diabetes, high blood pressure, and obesity.

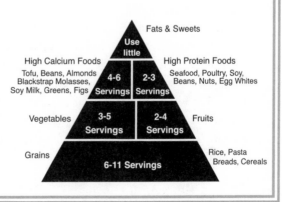

TRIGGER FOODS—WARNING! EAT AT YOUR OWN RISK

The most difficult foods for the body to digest are fats, meats, and dairy products. As a result, they are the most powerful IBS triggers, and you must strictly limit or, preferably, eliminate altogether these foods from your diet. Will this require an enormous change in the way you eat? Probably. But it is a change for the better, and we will walk together through the steps needed to make this change as easily and deliciously as possible.

I sympathize tremendously with people when they are told of the dietary changes they need to make to control their IBS. At first glance these changes can seem over-whelming and just too difficult, as by nature most of us are resistant to any great trans-formations of our lives. It is almost always easier not to alter a habit, simply because inertia takes less effort than action.

However, I really cannot stress enough that the changes in diet required for IBS do not equal deprivation. You will not be expected simply to give up all the foods you love and offered a tasteless starvation diet in return. These changes are in fact a terrific oppor-tunity for a better life, as you can easily learn how to eat safely for IBS without giving up an ounce of flavor, fun, favorite restaurants, or delicious home cooking. It is simply a matter of substitution, of replacing trigger foods with safe choices. Remember that the only thing you're really giving up here is the constant worry and dread of attacks, as well as the pain and agony they cause.

Please note that individual tolerances for IBS trigger foods may vary. The following list is comprehensive and should include all potential dietary sources of trouble. You may find through experimentation that you have a higher degree of tolerance for some of these foods than others.

Red Meat (Beef, Pork, Lamb, etc.)

Red meat is very high in fat, difficult to digest, and one of the strongest IBS triggers. Consumption of red meat is also clearly linked to numerous cancers, heart disease, osteo-porosis, diabetes, high blood pressure, gallstones, and foodborne illnesses,[21] so you will do your entire body a big favor by simply not eating it. Giving up red meat is probably the single greatest dietary change required to control IBS. It's up to you to decide if a Big Mac attack is worth the subsequent risk of an IBS attack. I know that it can take a lot of willpower to forego red meat if it is a favorite food. But I also know that most people who have suffered from IBS have gone without help for years, and have developed

[21] Barnard, Dr. Neal. The Medical Costs Attributable to Meat Consumption. Preventive Medicine, October 1995, Volume 24, Issue 6, 646–55.

indomitable wills and inner determination as a result. The lure of a steak pales in comparison to their strength of conviction.

Poultry Dark Meat and Skin

The fat content in poultry dark meat and skin makes them powerful triggers. Although skinless white meat is not a trigger, make sure to buy organic poultry only, as the drugs used in commercial poultry farms can have unknown effects on the GI tract.

Dairy Products

All dairy products—milk, butter, cheese, ice cream, and so on—and particularly those that are high fat, are very difficult to digest, *even if you are not lactose intolerant.* In addition to the fat and lactose, milk components such as whey and casein can also cause digestion problems. As a result, dairy is second only to red meat as an IBS trigger. As with red meat, this can be a tough category of food to avoid, but there is great news here. There are literally hundreds of low-fat soy, rice, and grain alternatives to dairy, for everything from cheese and butter to ice cream and chocolate milk. Start exploring your local health food store and you will be amazed. Dairy is honestly one of the easiest trigger foods to eliminate, because there are so many wonderful, healthier substitutes available that you will never have the chance to feel deprived.

Please note that there is no need to include dairy products in your diet to ensure adequate calcium intake. Dairy products offer a false sense of security to those concerned about osteoporosis, as numerous studies have found no benefits to dairy calcium regarding bone loss; in fact, increased dairy consumption has been shown to raise bone fracture risk.[22] The sulfate released from animal protein amino acid loads causes an over-acid condition in your body, due to the formation of uric acid and metabolic wastes. To remedy this situation your body needs to leach alkaline minerals, namely calcium and magnesium, out of your bones. These minerals are then excreted through urine. Due to this effect, when you eat dairy products your body will actually suffer a net calcium loss.[23]

---

[22] 1. Feskanich D, Willet WC, Stampfer MJ, Colditz GA. Milk, dietary calcium, and bone fractures in women: a twelve-year prospective study. Am J Public Health 1997; 87:992–7.

2. Cumming RG, Klineberg RJ. Case-control study of risk factors for hip fractures in the elderly. Am J Epidemiol 1994; 139:493–505.

3. Huang Z, Himes JH, McGovern PG. Nutrition and subsequent hip fracture risk among a national cohort of white women. Am J Epidemiol 1996; 144:124–34.

4. Cummings SR, Nevitt MC, Browner WS, et al. Risk factors for hip fracture in white women. N Engl J Med 1995; 332:767–73.

[23] Breslau, N. Relationship of animal protein-rich diet to kidney stone formation and calcium metabolism. J Clin Endocrinol Metab 66:140, 1988.

By age sixty-five, the average American woman who eats meat and dairy products has lost 35 percent of her skeleton; the average vegan woman has only lost 7 percent.[24] The best way to decrease the risk of osteoporosis is to reduce animal protein, sodium, and phosphate (found in soda pop) consumption,[25] increase fruit and vegetable intake,[26] exercise,[27] and add soy to your diet.[28] Studies show that the daily protein level commonly consumed by Americans (ninety grams or more) will cause more calcium to be lost from the body than can be absorbed from the gut, even when the person is consuming very high levels of calcium.[29] This is why populations around the world that eat diets loaded with animal proteins (the USA, England, Israel, Finland, Sweden, and so on) have high rates of osteoporosis, while people in countries who consume small amounts of animal proteins (meat and dairy), such as those in Asian and African countries, have strong bones and little osteoporosis. An African woman can have ten babies, nurse them for ten months each, and still have strong bones when she reaches the age of seventy, bones that are comparable to those of a twenty-year-old woman in America.[30] Eskimos, who daily consume 250 to 400 grams of animal protein and 2,200 mg of calcium from fish bone, have the highest incidence of osteoporosis of any population in the world.[31] In addition to osteoporosis, dairy products have been associated with breast, ovarian, and prostate cancers[32] as well as juvenile diabetes[33] and arthritis.[34] As with red meat, the healthiest diet will eliminate dairy products entirely.

[24] American Journal of Clinical Nutrition, March 1983.
[25] 1. Finn SC. The skeleton crew: is calcium enough? J Women's Health 1998 ; 7(1):31–6.
    2. Nordin CBE. Calcium and osteoporosis. Nutrition 1997; 3(7/8):664–86.
    3. Reid DM, New SA. Nutritional influences on bone mass. Proceed Nutr Soc 1997; 56:977–87.
[26] Tucker KL, Hannan MR, Chen H, Cupples LA, Wilson PWF, Kiel DP. Potassium, magnesium, and fruit and vegetable intakes are associated with greater bone mineral density in elderly men and women. Am J Clin Nutr 1999; 69:727–36.
[27] Prince R, Devine A, Dick I, et al. The effects of calcium supplementation (milk powder or tablets) and exercise on bone mineral density in postmenopausal women. J Bone Miner Res 1995; 10:1068–75.
[28] Endocrinology 1999 Apr; 140(4):1893–900.
[29] Breslau, N. Relationship of animal protein-rich diet to kidney stone formation and calcium metabolism. J Clin Endocrinol Metab 66:140, 1988.
[30] Marsh, A. Vegetarian lifestyle and bone mineral density. Am J Clin Nutr 43(3 suppl):837, 1988.
[31] Marsh, A. Vegetarian lifestyle and bone mineral density. Am J Clin Nutr 43(3 suppl):837, 1988.
[32] 1. Outwater JL, Nicholson A, Barnard N. Dairy products and breast cancer: the IGF-1, estrogen, and bGH hypothesis. Medical Hypothesis 1997; 48:453–61.
    2. Cramer DW, Harlow BL, Willet WC. Galactose consumption and metabolism in relation to the risk of ovarian cancer. Lancet 1989; 2:66–71.
    3. Chan JM, Stampfer MJ, Giovannucci E, et al. Plasma insulin-like growth factor-1 and prostate cancer risk: a prospective study. Science 1998; 279:563–5.
    4. World Cancer Research Fund. Food, Nutrition, and the Prevention of Cancer: A Global Perspective. American Institute of Cancer Research. Washington, D.C.: 1997.
[33] 1. Scott FW. Cow milk and insulin-dependent diabetes mellitus: is there a relationship? Am J Clin Nutr 1990; 51:489–91.

Egg Yolks

The high fat content in egg yolks makes them a powerful trigger. Although egg whites are a safe IBS food, make sure to buy organic eggs only as the drugs used in commercial poultry farms have unknown effects on the GI tract. Egg yolks can be eliminated from your diet quite painlessly. Omelets, quiches, and such can be made with all egg whites, as can most breads, cakes, and other desserts. This is one trigger food that you really won't miss at all—honest.

Fried Foods

There is no such thing as a low fat fried food, and as such, anything fried is an IBS trigger. I know how hard it is to give up foods like French fries and onion rings (believe me, I know), but there are a lot of great alternatives here. It's very easy to get crispy, crunchy results from oven baking or non-stick pan frying, with very little oil.

Coconut Milk

Although coconut is a fruit, it is extremely high in fat. Most of that fat is saturated, and thus poses additional health risks as well.

Oils, Shortening, Fats, Butter, Margarine

IBS does not distinguish between extra virgin olive oil and lard. Although monounsaturated fats (found in olive, canola, avocado, and nut oils) offer numerous general health benefits, and saturated fats pose serious health risks, all fats are IBS triggers, plain and simple.

Solid Chocolate

Solid chocolate has a very high fat content. Unsweetened cocoa powder, however, has no fat and is usually completely safe for baking. The good news here is that chocolate is a dessert, which means it's usually eaten in small quantities on a full stomach. Trigger foods can be much more tolerable under those circumstances. This means that you will probably be able to eat a little chocolate after a safe meal without risking an attack. I eat chocolate quite frequently in this manner with no problems at all. Hallelujah!

---

2. Karjalainen J, Martin JM, Knip M, et al. A bovine albumin peptide as a possible trigger of insulin-dependent diabetes mellitus. N Engl J Med 1992; 327:302–7.

[34] Skoldstam L, Larsson L, Lindstrom FD. Effects of fasting and lactovegetarian diet on rheumatoid arthritis. Scand J Rheumatol 1979; 8:249–55.

What's All this about Fiber?

One of the most troublesome pieces of advice routinely given to people with IBS is the dictate, "Eat more fiber!" It prompts the question—what kind of fiber?

Most people are never even told that there are actually two types of fiber. The term "fiber" in general refers to a wide variety of substances found in plants. Some of these substances can be dissolved in water ("soluble fiber"), while others do not dissolve ("insoluble fiber"). **Insoluble fiber** is "rough;" it passes intact through the intestines , which is why it is called "high-residue." It increases the frequency, water content, and looseness of bowel movements. Insoluble fiber, and particularly wheat bran, decreases the transit time of fecal matter in the GI tract. Although this has the crucial benefit of reducing the colon's exposure to carcinogens, thus inhibiting colon cancer development, it can also trigger severe attacks of pain and diarrhea in IBS sufferers. A study by Francis and Whorwell found that 55 percent of patients with IBS were made worse by wheat bran and only 10 percent found it helpful.[35]

Coffee, Regular and Decaffeinated

Coffee beans contain an enzyme that is such a powerful GI tract irritant it can cause abdominal cramps and diarrhea in people who do not even have IBS. In addition, the high amounts of caffeine in coffee can also trigger IBS attacks. Small amounts of instant coffee/espresso powder, used as an ingredient in cooking, are usually completely tolerable. If you can't open your eyes in the morning without that first cup of coffee, you probably already know you have a high tolerance level for the drink. Some people have no problems with it at all. If you're unsure, try waking up to a cup of peppermint, chamomile, fennel, or gingerroot tea instead.

Alcohol

This is a strong irritant to every organ in the digestive tract. You may find that your tolerance level for alcohol varies widely depending on the type of drink and whether the consumption is alone or with meals. You might have a very different reaction to a martini on an empty stomach than a glass of wine with dinner. If you have any doubts, it is safest not to drink at all. Small amounts of alcohol used for flavor in cooking are usually quite safe.

Carbonated Beverages

The carbonation in soda pop and mineral water can cause bloating and abdominal cramps, and the artificial sweeteners found in diet sodas can compound the problem. The high amount of caffeine in some sodas is also a trigger. Try getting in the habit of drinking herbal teas or still water instead.

[35] Francis CY and Whorwell PJ. Bran and the irritable bowel syndrome: time for reappraisal. Lancet 1994; 344: 19–4.
[36] Dr. David L. Katz, Yale School of Medicine, New Haven, Connecticut, presenting findings at the 1999 meeting of the American College of Nutrition, held in Washington, DC.

Artificial Sweeteners

All artificial sweeteners can cause abdominal cramps, pain, and diarrhea, although Sorbitol is the most notorious offender.

Artificial Fats

These products, particularly Olestra, can cause severe abdominal cramping and diarrhea.

INSOLUBLE FIBER—HOW CAN HEALTHY FOODS HURT YOU?

Insoluble fiber (high residue foods), although crucial for good health, can be a powerful IBS trigger. It needs to be incorporated into your diet in the largest quantities possible, but with great care. *Insoluble fiber should never be eaten alone or on an empty stomach.*

Remember that it is much better to have a wide variety of insoluble fiber foods in small amounts than not to eat any at all. You are also likely to find that your tolerance for insoluble fiber will increase if you are consistently eating it, even in tiny portions. However, it's important to note that individual tolerances vary. The following list is comprehensive and should include all potential insoluble fiber sources of trouble for a hyperactive colon; you may have a degree of tolerance for some of these foods and absolutely none for others. IBS is a highly personalized problem, so you will need to learn your own food tolerances and work around them.

Raw fruits, raw vegetables, raw greens, raw sprouts, and seeds (including those from fresh fruits or vegetables), are all very high in insoluble fiber. Be particularly careful with fruits and vegetables that have tough skins or hulls such as blueberries, cherries, apples, grapes, peas, corn, bell peppers, celery, and so on. It helps tremendously to peel and cook these fruits and vegetables until

Soluble fiber, in contrast, is "smooth," very low-residue, and soothing to the digestive tract. It absorbs excess water in the colon, forming a gel that pushes through impacted fecal matter, and it stabilizes and regulates intestinal contractions. In this manner it helps prevent the painful spasms and relieve *both* the diarrhea *and* constipation of IBS.

Soluble fiber also lowers LDL ("bad") blood cholesterol levels and the resultant risk of heart disease, helps prevent colon cancer, and improves glycemic control in diabetics by slowing the digestion of carbohydrates and the subsequent release of glucose into the blood. In addition, soluble fiber may help prevent blood vessel constriction and the formation of free radicals (both risk factors for heart attacks) by slowing the absorption of fat and carbohydrates into the bloodstream.[36]

Acacia Tummy Fiber, **Benefiber**, and **Citrucel** are all soluble fiber, and can be extremely helpful when taken daily (make sure they are *not* the sugar-free varieties, which have artificial sweeteners in them, and can trigger attacks). *Be aware that although some of these products are marketed as laxatives, technically they are not—they actually help treat and prevent diarrhea as well as constipation.* Soluble fiber alone has this remarkable ability to normalize colonic activity from either extreme.

For IBS, soluble fiber is also helpful because it fills the colon with bulk, helping to keep the GI muscles gently stretched around a full colon as opposed to tightly clenched around an empty colon.

Foods that are naturally high in soluble fiber include oatmeal, pasta, rice, potatoes, French or sourdough bread, soy, and barley. These starchy foods are also high in complex carbohydrates, which are an important source of readily accessible fuel for energy. Nuts, beans, and lentils are also good sources of soluble fiber but should be treated with care, as nuts are high in fat and both lentils and beans contain some insoluble fiber.

Soluble fiber should *always* be the first thing you eat on an empty stomach, and it should form the basis of every snack and meal. Your goal is to keep your colon consistently stabilized by providing it with a regular supply of soluble fiber.

tender, as this makes their fiber content dramatically less likely to trigger attacks. It is also a healthy habit to routinely incorporate fruits and veggies as secondary ingredients in recipes with soluble fiber foods as the main ingredients. If possible, buy organic produce only, as the chemical pesticides and herbicides used on fruits and vegetables can have adverse health effects.

Two categories of fruits and vegetables, those that are *acidic* and *sulfur-containing*, require extra precautions. **Citrus juice and cooked tomatoes** have very high acidity levels, which can cause GI distress, so they must be eaten with care. Incorporate them into meals (or drinks served with meals) with a high soluble fiber content, and don't eat them on an empty stomach. They must not be eliminated from your diet altogether, however, as they contain crucial vitamins and anti-oxidants. Tomatoes are also very high in lycopene, which prevents some forms of cancer.

Garlic, onions, leeks, broccoli, cauliflower, cabbage, and Brussels sprouts, though among the most nutrient-packed of all vegetables, can also pose problems. In addition to their high amounts of insoluble fiber, all contain sulfur compounds, which produce gas in the GI tract and can thus trigger attacks. As with other vegetables, cook these until tender, combine them with soluble fiber, and don't eat them when your stomach is completely empty—but do make sure and eat them.

An easy rule of thumb for all fruits and vegetables is to ask how easily "mashable" they are, as this will give you a quick gauge of their insoluble fiber content. Bananas, steamed sweet potatoes, mangoes, and applesauce are all very easy to mash, and thus safe to eat. Spinach leaves, bean sprouts, and kernel corn are not "mashable" at all, and thus need to be eaten quite carefully. Again, cooking your fruits and vegetables is of great help—just think of the difference between raw and cooked celery and you'll see what I mean.

To incorporate raw fruits and veggies into your diet, peel and eat them in small quantities (just two or three bites) finely chopped, as additions to high soluble fiber foods such as French breads, pastas, rice, and so on. It should also help to eat them toward the end of a meal. This is especially important when it comes to green salads. Eating them, as is customary in America, on an empty stomach at the beginning of lunch or dinner, is likely to trigger an attack. Eating them at the end of a high soluble fiber meal is typically quite safe. For fruit salads follow the same guidelines. At breakfast have a bowl of oatmeal or toasted French bread first, then the fruit, and at lunch or dinner have the fruit for dessert.

Remember that color is a good way to tell what types of nutrition fruits and vegetables offer; if you are completely intolerant of one try a same-color substitution. For example, if you can't eat cantaloupes, try mangoes. In my case, I can tolerate cabbage much more easily than lettuce though I don't know why.

Whole wheat and wheat bran are extremely high in insoluble fiber, and foods such as whole-wheat breads and cereals need to be eaten with great care. For a daily staple, French and sourdough breads are safe, but whole-wheat breads are not. Whole-wheat breads are more nutritious, because the outer coating of bran on the grain has not been removed as is the case in white breads. However, this bran is also very high in insoluble fiber, and can thus trigger attacks. For this same reason wheat bran cereals are not as safe a choice as rice, corn, or oat varieties are. Does this mean you should never eat whole-wheat bread or wheat bran cereal? It most emphatically does not. As with fruits and vegetables, the more whole grains you can eat the better. It cannot be stressed enough that overall good health is dependent on insoluble fiber. However, whole wheat and wheat bran need to be eaten just as carefully as green salads. Do not eat them on an empty stomach, in large quantities, or without soluble fiber foods.

Whole nuts can be high in insoluble fiber, and they are always high in fat. Although this fat is monounsaturated and lowers your risk of heart disease, it is still an IBS trigger. Like other insoluble fiber foods, nuts are crucial for good health, but must be eaten carefully. Finely grinding nuts and incorporating them into recipes with soluble fiber is a very safe way to eat them. Small amounts of nut butters on toasted French or sourdough bread are usually very tolerable as well.

Popcorn is full of hard kernels that are pure insoluble fiber. There is no great nutritional value to popcorn so it can simply be eliminated from your diet. I realize this may make movies a lot less fun, but having to bolt from a theater for the bathroom halfway through a film is a worse alternative. Sneak some pretzels or baked potato chips into the theater instead, and console yourself with the thought that you'll actually get to see the end of the movie if you bypass the popcorn concession stand.

Fresh fruit juices, especially apple, prune, and grape, can trigger cramps and diarrhea. Fruit juices in general should be avoided on an empty stomach. Cranberry juice is usually a safe choice.

Rhubarb, prunes, figs, licorice are all natural laxatives. As with fresh fruits in general, you may be able to incorporate these foods safely into recipes with soluble fiber. Just beware that they pose additional risks.

SPICE UP YOUR LIFE

You do *not* have to forego flavor and live on bland foods to avoid IBS attacks. Many people with IBS have been given this impression, but it is completely untrue. In fact, many typical bland foods—custards, puddings, warm milk, and so on—are major triggers due to their high fat and dairy content. On a related note, the real problem with spicy foods is that they are usually very greasy (chili, tacos, Sloppy Joes, curries) and often meat-based. It is their high fat content that causes problems, not their seasoning. Hot chili peppers such as cayenne, jalapeño, habanero, and so on, can cause GI distress in some people, but herbs and spices as a whole are not triggers for IBS. In fact, many herbs and spices, including ginger, mint, caraway, fennel, and chamomile, actually aid digestion. There is no limit on flavor when it comes to safe foods for IBS, so feel free to season your recipes any way you like.

ON A SWEET NOTE

One of the best things about the IBS diet is that it requires no restriction of sugar, which means that lots of luscious desserts are yours for the baking. This does not mean that sugar should become a main component of your diet, of course. Sugar has zero nutritional value and is nothing more than a simple carbohydrate with lots of empty calories. It should be used in moderation for general good health, and desserts should be limited to small portions following nutritious meals.

However, the fantastic thing about sugar is that it is most definitely not a trigger. It contains no insoluble fiber, no fat, no caffeine, no alcohol, and has no stimulant or irritant effect on the GI tract whatsoever. This is important to note, because some people with IBS find that they feel better when they eliminate sweets from their diet, and they then mistakenly assume that sugar must have been the underlying culprit. This isn't true—the real trigger in most desserts is fat. Butter, cream, egg yolks, shortening, solid chocolate, and whole milk form the basis of most traditional desserts, from cakes to cookies to ice cream. None of these foods are safe for IBS. So how can you enjoy traditional sweets? Easily and deliciously!

Desserts are among the simplest recipes to modify, and there are very few sweets that can't be made perfectly safe for IBS. Luscious creations are achieved with quite minor kitchen sleights-of-hand: cocoa powder replaces solid chocolate; soy and rice milk make perfect alternatives to dairy; two egg whites replace each whole egg; applesauce can reduce the amount of oil; and, incredibly, tofu can be whipped into fantasy desserts that are not only spectacularly delicious but positively healthy. These effortless substitutions are all it takes to have your cake and eat it too!

WHAT IF I'M A VEGETARIAN?

Well, first of all give yourself a richly deserved pat on the back. Vegetarianism is finally receiving due acknowledgment as the all-around healthiest diet possible. Vegetarians have lower heart disease, cancer, diabetes, osteoporosis, arthritis, and obesity risks, not to mention longer life expectancies.[37] But—is vegetarianism compatible with an IBS diet? Absolutely. In fact, the primary IBS dietary strategies (high soluble fiber/low fat) are, by nature, fundamentally vegetarian. You'll still need to eat insoluble fiber with great care, but you can easily substitute additional soy foods, beans, lentils, or nuts for seafood and poultry. For baking, egg white replacements are available at health food stores or through the Directory of Resources. I find myself becoming a stricter vegetarian each year and will probably end up completely vegan. The evidence is mounting that this is simply the healthiest diet possible. So if you're interested, by all means go veggie!

[37] Barnard ND, Nicholson A, Howard JL. Medical costs attributable to meat consumption. Preventive Medicine, October 1995, Volume 24, Issue 6, 646–55.

Strategy, Strategy, Strategy

∞

Question—What is the single most important principle to eating for IBS?
Answer—Organize every meal along the lines of easily tolerated,
high soluble fiber staples.

FRENCH OR SOURDOUGH bread, pasta, rice, potatoes, fat-free flour tortillas, baked corn chips (Tostitos), pita bread, oatmeal, soy foods, polenta, and so on, must form the foundation of every meal and snack. Think of vegetables, fruit, seafood, beans, lentils, nuts, egg whites, and chicken breasts as secondary ingredients to be used in smaller quantities for flavor.

TIPS, TRICKS, AND HELPFUL HINTS FOR EATING AND COOKING

- Eat soluble fiber first whenever your stomach is empty.
- Chew thoroughly. This will help prevent you from eating too fast and swallowing air, which can cause problems.
- Eat at a leisurely pace—if you must eat in a hurry, serve yourself half portions. Remember that the first stage of digestion occurs in your mouth, as saliva begins to break down food. The less you rush this process the better.

- Eat small portions of food, and eat frequently—the emptier your stomach is, the more sensitive you will be.
- Avoid eating large amounts of food in one sitting as this can trigger an attack.
- Avoid ice-cold foods and drinks on an empty stomach. Cold makes muscles contract, and your goal is to keep your stomach and the rest of your GI tract as calm as possible.
- Avoid chewing gum, as it causes you to swallow excess air, which can trigger problems.
- Drink fresh water constantly throughout the day (not ice cold). Limit the amount of water or other fluids you drink with your meals, as this can inhibit digestion.
- Eat green salads—tiny portions, with nonfat dressing—at the end of the meal, not the beginning (tell people you're French).
- Peel, skin, chop, and cook fruits and vegetables; lightly mash beans, lentils, corn, peas, and berries. Finely chop nuts, raisins and other dried fruits, and fresh herbs. Nuts in particular can be quite tolerable when finely ground. To keep dried fruit from sticking to your knife when chopping, spray the blade with cooking oil first.
- Use only egg whites (two whites can substitute for one whole egg), and try to buy organic.
- You can almost always reduce the amount of oil called for in recipes by at least ⅓.
- Use non-stick pans and cooking spray, as this will dramatically lessen the amount of oil you cook with. Remember, with IBS the less fat the better, period.

THINK SUBSTITUTION, NOT DEPRIVATION

- Substitute soy, rice, almond, or oat milk for all dairy milk (check the ingredients to be sure there is no added oil). Try a wide variety of brands and flavors as the difference in taste can be dramatic. Some brands are truly wretched and some are delicious. My favorite is VitaSoy lite vanilla. It's helpful to keep two types of soy/rice milk on hand: unsweetened for cooking and vanilla for drinking.
- Use soy or rice substitutes for cream cheese, sour cream, ice cream, and other dairy products (check the ingredients to be sure the items are low-fat).
- Many meat-based recipes such as tacos, Sloppy Joes, chili, and so on, can be easily adapted to IBS guidelines by substituting textured vegetable protein (TVP, a soy food available in health food stores) for the ground beef. Simply eliminate

the cooking oil and season the TVP as you would the meat. When well prepared most people honestly can't taste the difference. In addition, there are many vegetarian cookbooks available that replicate traditional American homestyle recipes with vegan substitutes for the dairy and meat ingredients. Try out several of these books from your local library and buy your favorites.

- Find a well-stocked local health food store and try a wide variety of vegan versions of deli meat, hot dogs, burgers, chicken wings, and so on. There are tasty versions of just about every fast food and junk food on the market—just check the ingredients for a low fat content.
- Use only fat-free salad dressings, mayonnaise, and so on.
- Substitute cocoa powder for solid chocolate.
- Use a small amount of blended, silken lite tofu to thicken soups, sauces, or shakes.
- If you have a weakness for a particularly deadly food (mine's cheesecake), try slowly eating just one to two measured tablespoons after a satisfying meal of high soluble fiber foods. I've found this to be a pretty foolproof method for occasionally treating myself.
- Watch out for hidden fat in seemingly safe foods: biscuits, scones, pancakes, waffles, restaurant French toast, crackers, mashed potatoes, and store-bought dried (usually fried) bananas.
- Explore ethnic markets. Asian grocery stores frequently carry fat-free noodles, dumplings, and snacks made with rice, bean paste, seafood, or tofu. Indian markets have nonfat crispy lentil wafers, special rice varieties, and many low fat vegetarian curries. Some things may sound unusual but they're worth a try. Most are delicious, healthy, and safe.

POWDERS, PILLS, AND POTIONS

- Take Acacia Tummy Fiber, Benefiber, or Citrucel (*not* sugar-free) every day. This may be the single greatest aid you'll ever find for controlling IBS.
- Carry Fibercon capsules (soluble fiber in a pill form) with you to have on hand when you unexpectedly have to wait too long between meals or eat at a restaurant. Take two pills with a large glass of water. Fibercon in general is not as effective as soluble fiber powders, but it is easier to carry in your purse or pocket and does provide a measure of protection in emergency situations.
- Peppermint is a smooth muscle relaxant, and can be very helpful in preventing/relieving IBS spasms. I consider it a wonder drug. Try drinking lots of

strong, hot mint tea throughout the day. It's inexpensive to make your own with dried peppermint leaves from bulk spice counters at health food stores. You can also try peppermints such as Altoids. I swallow them whole with meals as I would a prescription anti-spasmodic pill. You may wish to try Tummy Tamers, a brand of enteric-coated peppermint oil capsules, that are available in health food stores and pharmacies, or over the Internet (see Directory of Resources). They're perfectly legal and do not require a prescription. The directions state to take the capsules either on an empty stomach between meals or right before you eat a meal, so try both methods. However, be careful if you have GERD (Gastroesophageal Reflux Disease) or suffer from heartburn as mint in any form can worsen these symptoms.

- Take a multi-vitamin, multi-mineral supplement everyday. An additional 1,500 mg of calcium daily may also help, as calcium plays a critical role in regulating muscle contractions; it also has a constipating effect. In particular, Caltrate and Caltrate Plus have had spectacular results for many people. Women taking extra calcium may want to consider an iron supplement, as calcium can block the absorption of iron from foods and lead to anemia (take the calcium and iron supplements at different times of the day). Do *not* take antacids containing calcium, as all antacids have a laxative effect.

- Acidophilus (available as capsules) can normalize gastrointestinal flora, and may help prevent diarrhea in some people. It's especially beneficial if you are taking antibiotics. Acidophilus is widely available at drug stores and health food stores.

BE ACTIVE! BUT REST WHEN YOU NEED TO

- Try to be in motion after each meal. Go for a short, leisurely stroll around the block. Climb up and down a few flights of stairs at work. If you're at home, simply doing the dishes and cleaning up immediately after a meal should help. If you're at work, try to do things you can accomplish while standing. The point is to not become immobile on a full stomach, particularly while sitting down (and *never* lying down). You want to be gently active.

- Try to get thirty to sixty minutes of moderate aerobic exercise every day. Exercising regularly will help your whole body function better.

- Daily practice of yoga, meditation, or tai chi can significantly reduce stress-related attacks

- IBS hypnotherapy tapes have produced great results in some people (see Directory of Resources).

- Make sleep a priority. When you're tired your body simply cannot function properly, and this makes you more susceptible to attacks. In addition, sleep loss markedly decreases your ability to handle stress, and stress is a universal trigger. Try to take every opportunity you have to catch up on sleep by taking regular naps, setting an earlier weekday bedtime, and sleeping in on weekends.

FAST EASY FOODS

Fast food doesn't mean junk food. You can easily make yourself a quick, delicious snack or meal without spending a lot of time in the kitchen. More important, you can enjoy the following fast foods without the risk of spending a lot of time in the bathroom. So give yourself a treat while still treating yourself right.

- Chicken dip sandwiches (like a roast beef French dip—but make with toasted French rolls, shaved roasted chicken breast from the deli, and dip in hot fat-free chicken broth). Try to buy organic chicken.
- Tuna with nonfat mayo, finely diced onion and celery, on fat-free crackers.
- Lox and a smidgen of soy cream cheese on toasted bagels with thinly sliced red onions.
- Plain boiled prawns or crab legs with homemade cocktail sauce.
- Baked corn chips (Tostitos) with homemade salsas and bean dip.
- Homemade pizza snack mix.
- Homemade honey-glazed snack mix.
- Cold sweetened cereals such as Honeycomb or Corn Pops to snack on dry for dessert (check the ingredients for fat where you least expect it).
- Make a 9" x 13" pan of Rice Krispies treats with just 2 TB canola oil, extra cereal, and don't grease the pan.
- Heat a bowl of leftover rice with soy/rice milk, top with honey, cinnamon, and a diced mango or banana.
- Make a bowl of Cream of Wheat, Cream of Rice, or oatmeal, topped with brown sugar and a little sliced banana or mango.

WHAT TO EAT WHEN YOU CAN'T EAT ANYTHING

We've all been there. There are some days when it seems like everything you eat triggers an attack. When this happens, you need to give your body a break and stick to the safest foods possible.

- French or sourdough bread (not whole wheat or multi-grain).
- Toasted plain bagels.
- Toasted plain English muffins.
- Pretzels (salted or unsalted).
- Fat-free saltines.
- Angel food cake (homemade or from a mix).
- Fat-free fortune cookies.
- Arrowroot crackers.
- Graham crackers.
- Cold fat-free cereal such as Corn Chex, Kix, Rice Chex, Rice Krispies, Honeycomb, or Corn Pops, eaten dry. At all costs avoid wheat bran, granola, and whole-wheat choices, as well as cereals with raisins, other dried fruits, or nuts.
- Bowl of Will's Dreamy Lemon Rice Pudding, made without raisins (page 80).
- Homemade dried bananas.
- Plain cooked pasta (not egg), sprinkled with a little garlic salt.
- Bowl of Cantonese jok rice porridge soup (page 149).
- Lots and lots of strong hot peppermint, chamomile, fennel, or gingerroot tea.

TRAVELING—HOW TO LEAVE YOUR WORRIES BEHIND

If you have IBS, you already know how difficult it can be to eat safely when you're away from home. It is very important that you take extra precautions with your diet when traveling, as your regular routine will be disrupted and safe foods may not always be easily available. The key here is to plan ahead and bring your own supplies.

- If you are flying, call the airline and request a vegan, Asian vegetarian, seafood, or low fat meal.
- Assume that the airline may lose your request, so bring bread, fat-free crackers, dry cereal such as Rice Chex, Kix, or Honeycomb, home-dried fruit, and bottled water in your carry-on luggage. Whenever I fly I devote one small flight bag entirely to food. Yes, other passengers look at me funny when I haul out my own in-flight meal, but at least I don't have to worry about being trapped in the bathroom at twenty thousand feet.
- Snack frequently so your stomach is never empty.
- Make sure you take a supply of Metamucil or Citrucel (again, not sugar-free).
- For overnight stays, bring along individual envelopes of instant oatmeal. You can

make the cereal in your hotel room with just boiling water, and stabilize your-self first thing in the morning.

MAKE ROAD FOOD GOOD FOOD

- For road trips, always assume that the restaurants along the way won't serve anything you can eat (most of them probably won't), and make it a habit to take enough food for the day with you.
- Pack a generous picnic of breads or baked corn chips (Tostitos), homemade dips such as salsas or hummus, a small amount of fresh fruit, shaved chicken breast deli meat or roasted chicken white meat without the skin, boiled peeled prawns, angel food cake, or fortune cookies.
- Bring plenty of bottled water or herbal ice teas.
- Invest in a sturdy, compact ice chest for perishable foods.
- Stop at grocery stores along the way and replenish your supplies as needed.

Traveling can be a lot of fun with picnic lunches, and it's an enormous relief to not have to worry about getting sick from greasy road food.

RESTAURANTS—THE GOOD, THE BAD, AND THE DEADLY

Many people with IBS have come to the conclusion, borne of much painful experience and intimate knowledge of restaurant bathrooms, that they cannot eat out safely. Happily, nothing could be further from the truth. Restaurants are far too much fun to give up, and IBS does not require avoiding all the good things in life. It certainly does-n't require depriving yourself of great food. It does, however, take a little knowledge and a few handy tricks to eat out safely.

- Avoid fast food restaurants altogether. IBS and McDonalds are not compatible.
- If you know you will be eating out, snack on a lot of French bread or fat-free crackers beforehand so your stomach isn't empty.
- Take Metamucil or Citrucel (not sugar-free) before leaving for the restaurant.
- Carry Fibercon capsules (soluble fiber in a pill form) with you at all times in case you have to eat out unexpectedly. You can simply swallow the capsules with a glass of water as soon as you reach the restaurant.
- Watch what you eat first—no green salad or cream-based chowder, no alcohol, coffee, or carbonated beverages, especially on an empty stomach.

- Fill up on the bread basket (no butter!).
- Watch out for hidden fat. Look for simply steamed or broiled seafood, or grilled chicken.
- Ask for all sauces on the side and make sure that the meal comes with rice or a plain baked potato.
- Remember that restaurants typically serve much larger portions than you eat at home, so divide the food on your plate in half and eat slowly. Make it a rule to always leave the other half of your food to take home—this will help keep you from overeating, which can trigger an attack.
- Ask the waiter if you're not sure about an item. Don't be afraid to make special requests. You can tell the waiter you are not being picky, but that you have food allergies. Don't feel obligated to explain to anyone in detail why you need to eat the way you do, and don't be afraid to make your needs known. It's better to be a fussy customer and annoy a waiter than to pass out from pain in the bathroom.
- Bring a list of troublesome foods with you if it helps you remember what to watch out for, and check menu descriptions carefully.

If you happen to find yourself in a restaurant where there is literally nothing on the menu you can safely eat (and at typical American restaurants this is fairly likely), *get up and leave*. This can be awkward and embarrassing, and it is tempting in these situations just to take a chance and order something that looks semi-safe. This is not worth the risk. You'll only suffer from embarrassment until you make it to the parking lot, and once you've safely escaped you'll be glad you left. If you are with a group of people and leaving is not an option, order some plain bread, baked potato, oatmeal, or a side of rice, get a cup of mint tea to help you relax, and simply explain to the others that you have food sensitivities and there is nothing on the menu you can tolerate. Then politely change the subject and console yourself with the thought that at least you will not be getting sick, and that you can find some suitable food as soon as you leave.

TRY SOMETHING NEW, SOMETHING DIFFERENT

When it comes to restaurants, I have to admit that I've pretty much given up on traditional American food altogether in favor of ethnic choices. It's simply too difficult to find restaurants that serve safe versions of American standbys. However, this not such a bad thing, as there are so many fabulous ethnic restaurants serving delicious foods that will not trigger attacks. I've found that Asian restaurants in particular can be lifesavers.

Give some new places a try and see what you think.

- Japanese: sushi (there are lots of kinds without raw fish if you're squeamish), broiled fish, broiled tofu, udon soup, soba noodles.
- Chinese: dim sum, steamed vegetable or seafood dumplings, mu shu vegetables or shrimp, stir-fried seafood, chicken, and vegetable or shrimp choices (ask that very little oil be used), order extra servings of steamed white rice. Many Chinese restaurants have a special menu section of "healthy choices" that are steamed and have no oil added.
- Thai: pad Thai noodles (without pork), steamed seafood, and noodle dishes.
- Vietnamese: shrimp or vegetable rice dishes, seafood noodle soups, sautéed chicken or seafood dishes with extra orders of rice.
- Indian restaurants are good for baked breads with chutneys, and tandoori seafood or vegetarian dishes. Be sure to ask the waiter to make sure there is no cream and little oil in what you order.
- Deli or soup and sandwich places are a good bet for turkey or chicken sandwiches with mustard (no mayo or lettuce), and low fat vegetable or chicken noodle soups.
- Italian and Greek restaurants can be difficult. They add generous amounts of olive oil to just about everything.
- French restaurants pose problems. They rely heavily on meat, cheese, and cream sauces.
- Mexican restaurants can be dangerous. The corn chips are fried and there is frequently lard in the tortillas and sauces, as well as cheese melted over everything.

CAN I STILL HAVE FUN AT MOVIES, PARTIES, COOKOUTS, AND AMUSEMENT PARKS?

You probably know from firsthand experience how very difficult it can be to eat safely in these situations. Once again, the key is to be prepared for problems and plan ahead. For movies, amusement parks, ball games, and so on, bring small bags of pretzels, baked potato chips (Lays), or fortune cookies. Think in terms of substitution, not deprivation. You know you can't have the corndog and Coke, but what about a soft pretzel with an herbal ice tea (regular, not diet)? Candy is typically a safe way to splurge on junk food—it's primarily (if not entirely) sugar, and while this is hardly a health food it is not a trigger for IBS. Just avoid solid chocolate, coconut, and nuts, and look for mints, cotton candy, gumdrops, jelly beans, hard candies, and other fat-free choices. Eat a good meal right before leaving for these events, and have firm plans to head straight to a nearby restaurant (one with lots of safe menu choices) immediately afterwards. Remember that if there isn't anything safe to eat in these situations, you are better off eating nothing than eating the wrong thing.

For parties and cookouts take control of the situation ahead of time by phoning the host and explaining that you have a lot of food intolerances. Volunteer to bring several menu items; the party-giver will appreciate the help and you can bring food that you know is safe. For casual gatherings consider: baked potato chips (Lays), baked corn chips (Tostitos), homemade dips or salsas, homemade breads or cakes, Arizona Iced Teas or home-brewed herbal iced teas, homemade pizzas or mini soft tacos with safe ingredients, Rice Krispies treats made with very little oil, or bags of safe dime store candy. For cookouts, remember that the key is substitution: grill marinated salmon or catfish fillets, or barbecue skinless organic chicken breasts instead of hamburgers; bring baked potato chips (Lays) instead of fried ones; serve lots of fresh crusty French bread; make a potato salad with fat-free mayonnaise and skip the hard-boiled egg yolks; bake an angel food cake for a strawberry shortcake, or make fruit sorbet, and forget the ice cream; have lots of herbal iced tea on hand instead of soda pop. If you are hosting the party, just make everything you cook a safe choice. No one will even realize you aren't serving the typical greasy junk food if everything you make is simply delicious. In fact, you will likely find that many guests prefer to eat healthier foods even when they don't have IBS.

A New Way to Live

∞

IBS REQUIRES A bit of work when it comes to dietary planning, but the peace of mind that results from reducing your risk of attacks is a powerful motivating force. It's important to concentrate on the fact that you now have the knowledge required to take control of this problem, and to know that you will gain confidence as you change your life for the better.

Realize that you must develop the ingrained habit of thinking carefully about what you will be eating each and every day. Accept the time and planning this outlook requires as an utter necessity for your health and happiness. With a little practice you can easily incorporate this mindset into your life; eventually diet planning will become an automatic function, and a fundamental part of your daily routine just like sleeping and eating. Many people with IBS already spend time every day worrying about their problem, afraid they will suffer a sudden attack and the stress of trying to deal with it. It is an empowering change to instead spend this time ensuring that the problem will be solved for the day by eating what will help and not hurt.

In order to routinely know in advance exactly what you will be eating the next day, it is crucial that you make your diet a priority in your life: have a designated day of the week to grocery shop, and specific times set aside throughout the week to cook. Have the next day's meals and snacks identified before you go to bed at night. It may help to make a list of exactly what you'll be eating the following day. Make sure you always have plenty of snack foods available at home and at work. Take regular inventories of your pantry and freezer and keep a generous supply of safe staples (breads, dry cereals such as Corn Chex, Rice Chex, Kix, Honeycomb, Corn Pops, fat free crackers, rice, pasta, home-dried bananas, soy/rice milk, mint tea, and so on) on hand at all times. Consider buying a rice cooker. They're inexpensive and foolproof, and it's very helpful to have a constant supply of cooked rice in the fridge. Your goal is to never be caught without something safe to eat. Have your meals and snacks mentally planned long before you are actually hungry.

Remember that IBS often runs in cycles. Once your body is working well it will tend to continue that way. Conversely, if you are having frequent attacks, you must break the cycle. Accept that you need to give yourself special attention, relax, and realize that you will have to limit your diet strictly for several days, with no exceptions. This may mean literally living on bread and water, but it is important to listen to your body and not worry or feel guilty about your diet at this time. If you need to skip work or school, or cancel appointments, so be it. Allow yourself to just stay home all day and rest. If you can go for a slow and easy walk outside, try to do so. If you can't, you can't. Get extra sleep, indulge yourself with good books, trashy television, or whatever else easily occupies your mind and relaxes you. Remind yourself that you will recover, your digestion will stabilize, and you will be able to become more active and expand your diet. Women who find that their IBS flares with menstruation might make a monthly habit of restricting their diets to the safest foods possible during the first few days of their period. This can help head off attacks altogether.

Realize that you are the only person who has to be happy with your diet. No one else needs to understand or approve of what you can and cannot eat. Don't worry about what others think—your health is more important than avoiding their criticism. Realize that the diet you grew up on, and the foods you were taught are good for you, may no longer provide a healthy life. Many of us were raised on bacon and egg breakfasts, burger and fries lunches, meatloaf dinners, and ice cream desserts. This diet may be typical for most Americans, but it is simply intolerable for people with IBS.

Make a habit of listening to your body, and try to head off trouble before it becomes severe. IBS is a highly personalized problem. What works for you may not work for others, and vice versa.

You will probably more often than not be offered concern and compassion if you simply tell people why your diet is limited, and give them a brief explanation of IBS. Employers, co-workers, friends, and family are frequently very supportive when they know about your problem. It can feel awkward, embarrassing, or just plain tiresome to have to explain a health problem to others, particularly if you are a private person, but the results are likely to be consistently positive, and you will end up with much less stress and worry as a result. Having said this, you may also occasionally have people doubt and even criticize your inability to eat certain foods, particularly since IBS sensitivities are not as clear cut as, say, food allergies. Your tolerance may depend not only on what you eat, but the time of day, the size of the portion, whether or not you're eating on an empty stomach, how much stress you're under, and so on. It can be hard for people to understand that you simply cannot go to Burger King for lunch or eat the hot dogs and potato chips they offer at their barbecue. This is not your preference; it is a medical necessity. You must come to realize that no matter how difficult it may be for others to accept what you tell them about your dietary needs, it is even more difficult for you to survive a severe IBS attack. You have to reach a point in your life where you simply don't care what other people think about how you need to eat. You do not have to look for their understanding or approval, and you should not eat foods that hurt you just to avoid questions or criticisms. After all, other people don't ask for your approval of the way they eat. Your diet and your health are your business, and you should eat the way you must to live happily. If other people have a problem with that, it is their problem—not yours. It is much better to be thought difficult than to be in pain.

IBS Kitchen Essentials

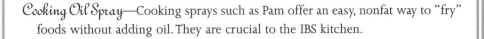

Cooking Oil Spray—Cooking sprays such as Pam offer an easy, nonfat way to "fry" foods without adding oil. They are crucial to the IBS kitchen.

Egg Whites—One of the fundamental strategies of IBS cooking is the substitution of two egg whites for one whole egg, thus eliminating the egg yolk, which is a trigger. If possible, buy organic eggs, as the hormones and other drugs used in commercial poultry have unknown effects on the GI tract. If you prefer, you may buy pasteurized egg whites in a carton (such as Egg Beaters), available in the dairy section of grocery stores, or use an egg white powder (such as Just Whites), available in the baking section of grocery stores, so you don't have to use up or throw out leftover egg yolks.

French and Sourdough Bread—These are truly indispensable staples of the IBS kitchen, because they are the perfect safe foundation for so many recipes. French toast, bread puddings, crostini and bruschetta, croutons for soups, bread salads, and more, all depend on French or Sourdough bread. Find a good local baker and make it a daily or weekly habit to stock up on several loaves, freezing extras so that you always have some on hand.

Herbal Teas—Peppermint, chamomile, fennel, and gingerroot can all be brewed into herbal teas that are extremely helpful for IBS. They relax the smooth muscles of the digestive tract, prevent abdominal cramping, relieve nausea, soothe upset stomachs, and are all-around terrific GI aids. Although you can buy ready-made tea bags in all of these varieties, it's a lot less expensive to buy the herbs in bulk and brew them in a tea strainer. Peppermint is available as leaves, chamomile as dried flowers, fennel as seeds, and gingerroot as a fresh root. All can be found at health food stores, some grocery stores, and spice shops, or through the Directory of Resources. My favorite is peppermint, and I make it a habit to have several cups a day. I buy peppermint leaves by the pound—and no, I'm not kidding.

Non-Stick Cookware—Non-stick frying pans are essential to the IBS kitchen, as they let you cook foods without adding any additional oil. Non-stick baking pans are also very helpful, as they require just a little cooking spray to produce perfect, easily removed breads and cakes.

Noodles—Pasta of every variety (except egg) is a great staple. Keep your cupboard well stocked with standbys such as spaghetti and fettuccine, but try a variety of Asian noodles as well. Rice noodles, fresh and dried, come in all shapes and sizes and form the basis of many Thai and Vietnamese dishes. Udon, soba, somen, lo mein, and flat wheat noodles are great for Japanese and Chinese cooking. All are available at Asian markets or through the Directory of Resources.

Rice and Rice Cookers—Quite a few types of rice are nice staples for the IBS kitchen. Rose rice is a short grain, white, sticky rice that goes beautifully with many Asian foods and also makes wonderful rice puddings. Jasmine rice is a very fragrant, long-grain white rice that is also delicious with Asian recipes. Basmati rice is a flavorful, long-grain white or brown rice that is perfect for Middle Eastern or Indian dishes. Brown rice has a nutty flavor and is available in short, medium, or long grain varieties. A rice cooker is an extremely convenient, inexpensive piece of cookware that is indispensable to the IBS kitchen. It is foolproof, fast, and a great way to cook a batch of rice every few days so you're never in short supply.

Soy Milk, Rice Milk, Oat Milk, Almond Milk—These milks are among the most essential staples of the IBS kitchen. They can substitute for dairy in virtually any recipe. Try a wide variety of brands and flavors, because the difference in taste can be dramatic. It's helpful to keep two types of milk on hand: unsweetened for cooking, and vanilla for drinking. Health food stores typically have the widest selection of milks, but grocery stores and ethnic markets carry multiple brands as well. My favorite brand is VitaSoy.

Soy Cheese—Health food stores carry a wide variety of soy cheeses, from cream cheese to Parmesan to mozzarella. Check the labels carefully to be sure you're buying a vegan, low fat brand. I've had good luck with the Soymage brand.

Soy Sauces—There are dozens of different types of soy sauce available, and many are deliciously different from the standard Japanese soy sauce, such as Kikkoman, that Americans are used to. Mushroom soy sauce, Thai thin soy sauce, and sweet black soy sauce are all available at Asian markets or through the Directory of Resources. Once you've tried them you will never again go without, as they are a fast, easy, and safe way to add a nice splash of flavor to almost any recipe. The best brand for flavored soy sauces is Healthy Boy. For basic soy sauces try Kikkoman or Jen Mai.

Tempering Eggs—This technique allows you to incorporate egg whites into a hot mixture, such as pudding or custard, without scrambling them. You simply add few spoonfuls of the hot mixture to the beaten egg whites, whisking thoroughly, and then add the whites to the remaining hot mixture.

Toasting Nuts and Seeds—All nuts and seeds benefit from toasting, as it heightens their flavor and fragrance. Simply heat a heavy skillet (*not* non-stick) without oil over medium high heat, add the nuts or seeds, and toast until golden brown, shaking the pan frequently to prevent burning.

Tofu—Tofu is available in many varieties, from firm to soft to silken. The silken version is sold packaged in aseptic boxes, which may be kept at room temperature until opened. Tofu is commonly carried by grocery stores, health food stores, and Asian markets. Widely available brands are is Mori-Nu and Nasoya.

SPECIALTY INGREDIENTS

Black Bean Garlic Sauce—This very aromatic paste is used as the base for many Asian stir-fry and seafood recipes. It is used in small quantities to add a rich, strong flavor without fat or heat. It's available at some grocery stores, Asian markets, or see the Directory of Resources. The best brand is Lee Kum Kee.

Chili Garlic Paste—This bright red paste is available in the ethnic section of some grocery stores and at Asian markets. It is used *very* sparingly to add a jolt of flavor to many Asian dishes. The best brand is Lee Kum Kee.

Chipotle Peppers—Chipotle peppers are smoked, dried jalapeños used in very small quantities. They lend an incomparable smoky flavor to foods without adding much heat, and they really have no substitute. Small bags of whole or ground peppers are available at many supermarkets and Hispanic markets, or see the Directory of Resources. Grind whole chipotles to a powder in a spice or coffee grinder. An entire bag of chiles (easily a year's supply) can be ground at one time and stored in a glass bottle. They are truly worth the effort. Do not substitute canned chipotles in adobo sauce, as they have a different flavor and a much higher heat level.

Fish Sauce—This ingredient is essential to Thai and Vietnamese recipes. You can use either *nam pla* (Thai) or *nuoc mam* (Vietnamese), whichever you prefer. Fish sauce is available at Asian markets, in the ethnic section of some grocery stores, or through the Directory of Resources. Squid, Tiparos, and Healthy Boy are all good brands.

Red Onion or Shallot Flakes—These are available in small jars at Asian markets, and they lend an addictive flavor and crunch to stir-fries or salads. They are used in such small quantities that they add only a trace amount of fat.

Lemongrass—Fresh lemongrass stalks add a sweet, lemony note to Southeast Asian dishes. They have a very strong perfume but no acidity. Lemongrass comes in long stalks with tough outer leaves. To use, remove the outer layers until you reach the more tender inner core, and mince finely. Lemongrass is available in the produce section of some grocery stores, health food stores, and Asian markets.

Mirin—Mirin is sweet sake used in Japanese cooking. It's made from short-grain rice, glutinous rice, and distilled alcohol. The combination of alcohol and sugars gives mirin its distinctive flavor and sweetness, and imparts a sheen to foods when used as a sauce ingredient, as in teriyaki. Mirin is available in the ethnic section of some grocery stores, Asian markets, or through the Directory of Resources.

Miso—Miso paste is a fermented soybean product that is rich in phytoestrogens. It is also one of the few non-animal sources of vitamin B_{12}. It comes in several varieties, packed in small plastic containers, and is available in the refrigerated section of many grocery store produce sections, health food stores, or Asian markets. Miso will keep indefinitely in your refrigerator.

Orange Flower Water and Rose Water—Orange flower water and rose water lend a very subtle, exotic, and distinctive perfume to breads and desserts. They are essential to many Middle Eastern and Indian recipes. They are available at Indian or Middle Eastern Markets, spice shops, baking or pastry supply shops, or see the Directory of Resources.

Pepitas—Pepitas are Mexican green pumpkin seeds. Toasting them heightens their flavor, and finely grinding them makes them very tolerable. They are nutritious and lend a unique, earthy flavor to sauces. They are available at many health food stores, specialty markets, Hispanic or Indian markets, or through the Directory of Resources.

Roasted Tomatoes—Roasting tomatoes gives them a sweet, smoky flavor. Simply place the tomatoes in a broiling pan and broil as close to the heat source as possible until the skins are black and blistered. Turn the tomatoes occasionally so they roast evenly. Let them cool then slip off the skins.

Sesame Oil—Sesame oil gives a rich, nutty flavor to dishes and is available in the ethnic section of many grocery stores, at health food stores, and Asian markets. Make sure you buy the dark brown variety made from toasted seeds, as it is much more flavorful. A tiny bit of sesame oil goes a very long way.

Surimi—Surimi is imitation crab made from white fish and seasonings. It is widely available in the seafood section of grocery stores or at Asian markets.

Tamarind—Tamarind is a sour fruit used in puréed form in many Southeast Asian and Indian recipes. The easiest way to use it is to buy the fruit concentrate, sold in small jars. The best brand is TamCon. TamCon is available at Asian, Hispanic, or Indian markets, or see Directory of Resources.

Toasted Sesame Seeds—Toasted sesame seeds are much more flavorful than untoasted varieties. They are visibly darker than the white, untoasted seeds. They are available in the ethnic section of grocery stores or at Asian markets. You can toast your own seeds by following the directions for toasting nuts, above.

Textured Vegetable Protein—TVP is a dehydrated, de-fatted, flavorless soy product sold in large flakes. It is reconstituted with liquid and seasonings to form a ground meat substitute. As odd as it sounds, TVP makes truly delicious and totally safe veggie burgers, chili, tacos, and a wide range of other recipes that call for ground meat. It can convincingly substitute for ground beef, pork, chicken, or seafood. Because it has no flavor on its own, it can be seasoned however you wish, and it will absorb the tastes of the foods it is cooked with.

RECIPES

∞

ALL RECIPES INCLUDED in this book have a nutritional analysis per serving of calories, protein, percentage of calories from protein, carbohydrates, percentage of calories from carbohydrates, total fat, percentage of calories from fat, saturated fat, cholesterol, sodium, and total dietary fiber. (Analysis provided by NutriBase '98 Nutrition Manager software, approved for use by licensed dieticians.)

BEVERAGES

∞

*T*HE ALL-AROUND best beverage for IBS is a cup of hot, strongly brewed peppermint, chamomile, fennel, or gingerroot tea. The worst is a three-way tie between coffee, alcohol, and soda pop. Are there any other choices? You bet there are. Blended beverages are a wonderful way to eat fresh fruit, as the insoluble fiber in foods like strawberries and peaches is much less of a trigger when it's finely puréed. Ingredients like ginger and fennel are very soothing to the GI tract, and lend themselves deliciously to a wide variety of teas. Creamy drinks are a breeze with soy milk or tofu, and additions such as bananas and almonds add lots of soluble fiber. Remember that it's safest to drink fresh fruit beverages with meals, and that ice-cold liquids can cause problems on an empty stomach, but feel free to enjoy the hot teas at any time.

HIGH-ENERGY BANANA CAROB BREAKFAST SHAKE

∞

*B*reakfast in a glass! Fast, easy, and nutritious, this drink is a great start to any day. It's low fat, has high soluble fiber, and just happens to be perfectly delicious.

MAKES 1 SERVING (EASILY DOUBLED OR TRIPLED)

1 firm-ripe banana
1 organic egg white*
¼ cup vanilla soy or rice milk
2 tablespoons carob powder

Combine all ingredients in blender and purée until smooth, scraping down sides of blender with rubber spatula if necessary. Pour into a large glass and serve.

*If salmonella is a concern in your area you can substitute pasteurized egg whites, available in the dairy section of most grocery stores (such as Egg Beaters).

NUTRIENT ANALYSIS PER SERVING:
Calories (kcal) 197.55

Protein (g) 7.34	Calories from Protein 24.49	% Calories from Protein 12.40
Carbohydrates(g) 47.54	Calories from Carbohydrates 158.60	% Calories from Carbohydrates 80.28
Fat (g) 1.93	Calories from Fat 14.46	% Calories from Fat 7.32
Saturated Fat (g) 0.40	Total Dietary Fiber (g) 10.43	Sodium (mg) 69.09

STRAWBERRY-BANANA SMOOTHIE

∞

*T*his is a great breakfast shake to accompany a bowl of oatmeal or toasted sourdough English muffins. The banana adds soluble fiber, and the strawberries lend a luscious sweetness to the morning.

MAKES 2 SERVINGS

    1½ cups frozen strawberries, very slightly thawed
    ⅔ cup vanilla soy milk
    1 tablespoon honey
    1 large firm-ripe banana

Purée all ingredients in blender until smooth. Serve immediately.

NUTRIENT ANALYSIS PER SERVING:
Calories (kcal) 160.54

Protein (g) 3.46	Calories from Protein 12.55	% Calories from Protein 7.82
Carbohydrates(g) 36.27	Calories from Carbohydrates 131.59	% Calories from Carbohydrates 81.97
Fat (g) 2.01	Calories from Fat 16.40	% Calories from Fat 10.22
Saturated Fat (g) 0.31	Total Dietary Fiber (g) 5.06	Sodium (mg) 13.14

CHINESE GREEN TEA WITH HONEY

∞

*P*owdered green tea is widely available at health food stores and Asian markets, and is well worth a special trip. It brews to a brilliant shade of jade green, and has a delicate, slightly woodsy flavor. Green tea is very soothing in the morning or with Asian meals, and offers a terrific health bonus—the anti-oxidants it contains have been shown to lower several cancer risks.

MAKES I SERVING (EASILY DOUBLED OR TRIPLED)

I cup water
⅛ teaspoon Chinese green tea powder
I teaspoon honey

Heat water until hot but not boiling. Whisk in tea powder and honey with a fork until frothy. Serve hot.

NUTRIENT ANALYSIS PER SERVING:

Calories (kcal) 21.28		
Protein (g) 0.02	Calories from Protein 0.08	% Calories from Protein 0.36
Carbohydrates(g) 5.77	Calories from Carbohydrates 21.20	% Calories from Carbohydrates 99.64
Total Dietary Fiber (g) 0.01		
Sodium (mg) 0.28		

SOOTHING SWEET PEPPERMINT GREEN TEA

∞

This is my favorite breakfast tea, especially on chilly days. For stressful times it is the perfect drink to help you relax.

MAKES 6 SERVINGS

2 cups packed fresh mint leaves
½ cup granulated sugar
6 cups boiling water
1½ teaspoons green tea powder

Place all ingredients except the tea powder in a teapot, and stir to dissolve the sugar. Let steep 4 minutes, add the tea powder, and let steep 1 minute. Stir well. Strain mint leaves out of tea. Serve hot or chilled.

NUTRIENT ANALYSIS PER SERVING:
Calories (kcal) 195.28

| Carbohydrates (g) 50.48 | Calories from Carbohydrates 195.28 | % Calories from Carbohydrates 100.00 |
| Saturated Fat (g) 0.00 | Sodium (mg) 0.50 | |

SPRING BLOSSOM TEA

∞

This delicate, exceptionally fragrant tea is refreshing hot or cold and makes a perfect accompaniment to Thai or Vietnamese food. It's also delicious with chocolate desserts.

MAKES 1 SERVING

12 oz. purified or bottled water
1 teaspoon jasmine tea with blossoms*
½ teaspoon rosewater**
¼ teaspoon orange flower water**

Bring water to a boil. Add tea in a tea strainer; brew for 30 seconds. Add rosewater and orange flower water. Serve hot or chill for iced tea.

*Jasmine tea is available at many grocery stores, spice shops, tea shops, or Asian markets, or see Directory of Resources.

See **Specialty Ingredients (page 34)

NUTRIENT ANALYSIS PER SERVING:
Calories (kcal) 0

Protein (g) 0	Calories from Protein 0	% Calories from Protein 0
Carbohydrates (g) 0	Calories from Carbohydrates 0	% Calories from Carbohydrates 0
Fat (g) 0	Calories from Fat 0	% Calories from Fat 0
Saturated Fat (g) 0	Total Dietary Fiber (g) 0	Sodium (mg) 0

Indian Chai Milk Tea

∞

his is the safe version of a tea served at most Indian restaurants. The spices are exotic but subtle, and the soy milk gives a smooth creamy result without the risk of dairy.

MAKES 1 SERVING (EASILY DOUBLED OR TRIPLED)

CHAI MIX:

1 tablespoon whole cloves
1 tablespoon whole fennel seeds
1 tablespoon whole cardamom seeds (not in pods)
2 small cinnamon sticks, broken into small pieces

1 cup vanilla soy or rice milk
1 teaspoon honey

Stir together all chai mix ingredients. Add 1 tablespoon chai mix to soy milk and bring to a boil. Remove from heat and steep for 3 minutes. Strain and stir in honey. Store extra chai mix in an airtight container.

NUTRIENT ANALYSIS PER SERVING:
Calories (kcal) 102.13

Protein (g) 6.76	Calories from Protein 25.11	% Calories from Protein 24.59
Carbohydrates(g) 10.20	Calories from Carbohydrates 37.90	% Calories from Carbohydrates 37.11
Fat (g) 4.68	Calories from Fat 39.11	% Calories from Fat 38.30
Saturated Fat (g) 0.52	Total Dietary Fiber (g) 3.20	Sodium (mg) 29.68

RAINY DAY LEMON AND GINGER TEA

*T*he perfect tea for cold, dark nights, this drink will chase away the winter blues. It's ginger-spicy, sweet-tart, and soothing all at once, and I swear it even cures colds.

MAKES 3 SERVINGS (EASILY DOUBLED)

> 8" piece of thick fresh gingerroot, peeled and sliced into thin coins
> 3 cups water
> 1/4 cup honey
> 1/4 cup granulated sugar
> Zest of one lemon
> 1/2 cup fresh lemon juice

In a small saucepan combine all ingredients except lemon juice and bring to a boil, stirring until sugar is dissolved. Cover pan and remove from heat. Let steep 30 minutes. Add lemon juice, stir well, and strain into mugs. Tea may also be chilled and served cold.

NUTRIENT ANALYSIS PER SERVING:
Calories (kcal) 161.06

Protein (g) 0.24	Calories from Protein 0.88	% Calories from Protein 0.55
Carbohydrates(g) 43.57	Calories from Carbohydrates 160.18	% Calories from Carbohydrates 99.45
Total Dietary Fiber (g) 0.22	Sodium (mg) 1.70	

TART CRANBERRY, LIME, AND HONEY REFRESHER

∞

This is a fast and easy drink, chock-full of Vitamin C, and perfect with lunch or an afternoon snack.

MAKES 1 SERVING (EASILY DOUBLED OR TRIPLED)

1½ cups cranberry juice
Juice from ½ lime
2 teaspoons honey

Stir all ingredients together with a fork (to help dissolve the honey) in a large glass.

NUTRIENT ANALYSIS PER SERVING:
Calories (kcal) 268.75

Protein (g) 0.28	Calories from Protein 1.05	% Calories from Protein 0.39
Carbohydrates(g) 69.67	Calories from Carbohydrates 263.86	% Calories from Carbohydrates 98.18
Fat (g) 0.45	Calories from Fat 3.84	% Calories from Fat 1.43
Saturated Fat (g) 0.04	Total Dietary Fiber (g) 1.35	Sodium (mg) 8.81

MANDARIN GINGER ZINGERS

∞

*T*errifically comforting, this is a hot drink for any time of day or night. The ginger is very soothing to all types of digestive troubles.

MAKES 1 SERVING

> 1 cup fresh orange juice
> 1" chunk fresh gingerroot, peeled and roughly smashed with the flat side of a
>   heavy knife
> ½ cup water
> 1 tablespoon honey

Bring the first three ingredients just to a boil in a small saucepan. Remove from heat
and let steep for 2–3 minutes. Add honey, stir well, and strain into a glass.

NUTRIENT ANALYSIS PER SERVING:
Calories (kcal) 183.03
Protein (g) 1.99 | Calories from Protein 7.58 | % Calories from Protein 4.14
Carbohydrates(g) 44.76 | Calories from Carbohydrates 170.51 | % Calories from Carbohydrates 93.16
Fat (g) 0.58 | Calories from Fat 4.94 | % Calories from Fat 2.70
Saturated Fat (g) 0.08 | Total Dietary Fiber (g) 0.76

SUMMER PEACHY LEMONADE

∞

*T*his is probably my very favorite lemonade in the whole wide world. The peaches make it thick and frothy and add a note of sweet perfume to the tartness of the lemons. Serve this with a meal for a special summer treat.

MAKES 4 SERVINGS

> ½ cup fresh lemon juice
> ⅓ cup granulated sugar
> ½ cup water
> 4 cups frozen fresh peach slices, very slightly thawed

Combine all ingredients except the peaches in a blender and blend well. Slowly add the peach slices a few at a time and blend well after each addition. Pour into glasses and serve immediately with a meal.

NUTRIENT ANALYSIS PER SERVING:
Calories (kcal) 145.23

Protein (g) 1.31	Calories from Protein 4.76	% Calories from Protein 3.28
Carbohydrates(g) 38.15	Calories from Carbohydrates 139.20	% Calories from Carbohydrates 95.85
Fat (g) 0.15	Calories from Fat 1.26	% Calories from Fat 0.86
Saturated Fat (g) 0.02	Total Dietary Fiber (g) 3.52	Sodium (mg) 0.47

FRESH MINT-LEAF LEMONADE

∞

*F*or a pretty touch at a luncheon, bridal shower, or midsummer cookout, serve this lemonade chilled in clear glasses with ice cubes that have fresh flowers frozen within. Simply place a well-rinsed, homegrown, unsprayed edible flower blossom (miniature roses, rose petals, jasmine, violets, pansies, lavender) in each segment of an ice cube tray, fill halfway with water, and freeze. When frozen, fill the tray to the top with water and refreeze. Doing this in two steps will keep the blossoms completely encased in ice.

For an elegant snack serve this lemonade with English Teatime Shrimp and Watercress Finger Sandwiches (page175) and toasted slices of Sweet-Tart Orange Cranberry Bread (page 99).

MAKES 3 12-OZ. SERVINGS

> 1½ cups packed fresh mint leaves, washed, dried, and chopped
> 1 cup granulated sugar
> 1 cup water
> Juice of 3 lemons
> Purified or bottled water

Make a mint syrup by combining mint leaves, sugar, and water in a small saucepan. Heat and stir until sugar dissolves; bring to a boil and simmer until syrup reduces to about 1 cup. Chill. Strain syrup, pressing hard on solids and discarding mint leaves. Divide juice from lemons among three tall glasses; add ⅓ cup syrup (or to taste) to each glass to sweeten. Fill glasses with water, stir well, and add ice. Serve with meals.

NUTRIENT ANALYSIS PER SERVING:
Calories (kcal) 269.75

Protein (g) 0.18	Calories from Protein 0.68	% Calories from Protein 0.25
Carbohydrates (g) 70.66	Calories from Carbohydrates 269.07	% Calories from Carbohydrates 99.75
Total Dietary Fiber (g) 0.1	Sodium (mg) 1.14	

Mexican Cinnamon-Lime Horchata

∽

A horchata is a Mexican iced drink made from ground nuts, seeds, or rice. The high soluble fiber content of almonds makes this a safe drink, particularly because the nuts are so finely ground. This recipe is smooth, light, and refreshing, and offers a delicious accompaniment to many foods. For a sweet and soothing end to a hot summer day, pour a glass to enjoy after dinner as you sit on your front porch or stoop and watch the sun go down.

If you wish to double this recipe, make two separate batches or you will overfill your blender.

MAKES 4 SERVINGS

1 cup sliced almonds
2 cup boiling water
1 large cinnamon stick, broken into pieces
Grated zest from one lime
½ cup granulated sugar
2 cups crushed ice cubes

In a blender combine all ingredients except ice. Let sit for 15 minutes. Blend mixture on high speed for 3–4 minutes. Add ice and blend for 2 minutes.

Slowly pour mixture into a large pitcher through a fine mesh sieve or a double layer of dampened cheesecloth, pressing hard on solids to extract as much liquid as possible. Discard solids. Chill the filled pitcher until cold, and preferably overnight.

NUTRIENT ANALYSIS PER SERVING:
Calories (kcal) 303.71

Protein (g) 5.70	Calories from Protein 21.49	% Calories from Protein 7.08
Carbohydrates (g) 34.67	Calories from Carbohydrates 130.73	% Calories from Carbohydrates 43.04
Fat (g) 17.86	Calories from Fat 151.49	% Calories from Fat 49.88
Saturated Fat (g) 1.70	Total Dietary Fiber (g) 5.65	Sodium (mg) 4.49

VIRGIN STRAWBERRY DAIQUIRIS
∞

*T*hese daiquiris are summer in a glass—ruby-red, sweet, and luscious. During heat waves I can frequently be found sitting au naturel in front of a fan drinking entire pitchers. If you're serving guests who prefer their drinks sinful to virginal, add spiced rum to the daiquiris to taste. For a fabulous outdoor dinner combination, try them with Jamaican Chicken with Ginger Peach Chutney (page 202). And for best results do be sure to use frozen berries (you can freeze fresh berries, if you prefer).

MAKES 4 SERVINGS

   ½ cup Rose's lime juice
   ¼–⅓ cup granulated sugar
   Juice of half an orange
   4 cups frozen fresh whole strawberries, very slightly thawed

Combine all ingredients except the strawberries in a blender and blend well. Slowly add the strawberries a few at a time and blend well after each addition. Pour into glasses and serve immediately with a meal.

NUTRIENT ANALYSIS PER SERVING:
Calories (kcal) 127.95

Protein (g) 0.79	Calories from Protein 2.92	% Calories from Protein 2.28
Carbohydrates(g) 33.43	Calories from Carbohydrates 122.91	% Calories from Carbohydrates 96.06
Fat (g) 0.26	Calories from Fat 2.12%	Calories from Fat 1.66
Saturated Fat (g) 0.02	Total Dietary Fiber (g) 3.27	Sodium (mg) 8.17

APPETIZERS AND SNACKS

∞

I CONFESS, I PREFER snacks to meals, and I'd rather have a dinner of several different appetizers than one big entree. I don't feel guilty, though, because it's important for those of us with IBS to eat small amounts of food frequently. With so many safe and wonderful treats to snack on, it's a lot of fun, too. Toasted French bread, baked corn chips, and pitas form the perfect high soluble fiber basis for lots of delicious low fat dips, spreads, nibbles, and noshes. Baked potato chips, pretzels, and corn or rice cereals are fast, safe snack foods when you're on the run, but the following recipes are almost as easy and offer a wide variety of tasty, healthy options.

SMOKY BLACK BEAN DIP

∞

*T*his creamy, smoky dip is utterly irresistible. Beans are very high in soluble fiber and puréeing them makes the insoluble fiber of their skins very tolerable. Spread this dip on baked corn chips, flour tortillas, pita bread—it would make cardboard edible! I never make fajitas or burritos without my trusty black bean dip to accompany them. Even people who claim they don't like beans will rave about this recipe—it really is that good.

MAKES 4 SERVINGS. RECIPE EASILY DOUBLES.

> 1 15-oz. can of drained, rinsed black beans
>   (or 1½ cups cooked homemade black beans)
> 4 large cloves garlic, minced to a paste with dash salt
> ¼–½ teaspoon ground chipotle pepper (adjust to taste for heat)*
> 1 tablespoon fresh lime juice
> 1 tablespoon white vinegar or white wine vinegar
> ¼ teaspoon ground cumin
> 2 teaspoons ground chili powder
> 2 tablespoons soy cream cheese
>
> Baked corn chips (Tostitos) for serving

Add all ingredients to a food processor and blend until smooth. Fill a glass bowl with dip, cover, and microwave until hot, about 3–5 minutes. Serve with generous amount of baked corn chips.

*See **Specialty Ingredients** (page 34)

NUTRIENT ANALYSIS PER SERVING:
Calories (kcal) 111.58

Protein (g) 8.99	Calories from Protein 35.12	% Calories from Protein 31.48
Carbohydrates(g) 18.09	Calories from Carbohydrates 70.69	% Calories from Carbohydrates 63.35
Fat (g) 0.66	Calories from Fat 5.77	% Calories from Fat 5.17
Saturated Fat (g) 0.28	Cholesterol (mg) 1.70	Total Dietary Fiber (g) 5.69
Sodium (mg) 117.11		

MEXICAN CUMIN AND GARLIC REFRIED LENTILS

∞

*T*his recipe is a wonderful alternative to traditional fat-laden refried beans. Lentils are incredibly nutritious and loaded with soluble fiber. Try this spread with chips or as part of a Mexican meal.

MAKES 4 SERVINGS

I cup red lentils, washed, picked over, and drained
3 cups water
I teaspoon cumin
I teaspoon chili powder
I teaspoon garlic salt
I cup finely chopped onion
2 tablespoons olive oil
I large garlic clove, minced
I tablespoon fresh lime juice
2 tablespoons finely chopped fresh cilantro

Baked corn chips (Tostitos) for serving

In a medium saucepan combine lentils, water, cumin, chili powder, and garlic salt. Bring to a boil, whisking frequently with a metal whisk, and cook until smooth, about 40 minutes.

While lentils cook, sauté onion in oil in a large non-stick skillet until onions are golden. Add garlic and cook, stirring, five minutes. Add lentil purée and lime juice and combine well. Top with cilantro, and serve with baked corn chips.

NUTRIENT ANALYSIS PER SERVING:
Calories (kcal) 247.40

Protein (g) 12.70	Calories from Protein 49.11	% Calories from Protein 19.85
Carbohydrates(g) 33.08	Calories from Carbohydrates 127.88	% Calories from Carbohydrates 51.69
Fat (g) 8.10	Calories from Fat 70.42	% Calories from Fat 28.46
Saturated Fat (g) 1.13	Total Dietary Fiber (g) 6.25	Sodium (mg) 594.19

BRUSCHETTA WITH WHITE BEAN AND ALMOND DIP

∞

*T*his is a creamy, rich, and well-seasoned dip. The almonds and puréed beans form a silky base that you'd swear is high in fat, but of course it isn't. It is, however, full of flavor and soluble fiber.

MAKES 1½ CUPS, ABOUT 6 SERVINGS

⅓ cup almonds
15–16 oz. can white beans (or 1½ cups homemade beans), rinsed and drained
2 teaspoons fresh lemon juice
1 tablespoon extra-virgin olive oil
¼ cup plain soy or rice milk
2 tablespoons dried parsley
¼ teaspoon paprika
1 small garlic clove, mashed to a paste with ¼ teaspoon salt

Six large slices of horizontally sliced baguettes or rustic Italian bread, toasted

In a large ungreased frying pan (not non-stick) toast the almonds over medium high heat until lightly golden, shaking pan frequently. Cool. Add nuts and remaining ingredients to a food processor or blender and purée until smooth. Serve dip with toast slices.

NUTRIENT ANALYSIS PER SERVING:
Calories (kcal) 254.51

Protein (g) 10.20	Calories from Protein 40.03	% Calories from Protein 15.73
Carbohydrates(g) 37.23	Calories from Carbohydrates 146.15	% Calories from Carbohydrates 57.43
Fat (g) 7.74	Calories from Fat 68.33	% Calories from Fat 26.85
Saturated Fat (g) 0.99	Total Dietary Fiber (g) 5.98	Sodium (mg) 314.51

CRUNCHY GARLIC BRUSCHETTA WITH FRESH TOMATOES AND BASIL

ere's the perfect way to enjoy summer's bounty of garden-ripe tomatoes, with a crunchy garlic kick. It makes a quick safe snack or a great light lunch.

MAKES 1 SERVING (EASILY DOUBLED OR TRIPLED)

- 1 6" baguette, halved horizontally
- 1 large garlic clove, minced
- 1 teaspoon olive oil
- 1 medium ripe tomato, diced
- 2 tablespoons onion, diced
- 1 tablespoon finely shredded fresh basil leaves

Combine the garlic and olive oil, and spread evenly over baguette halves. Toast until golden brown. Combine tomato, onion, and basil, and spoon over bruschetta.

NUTRIENT ANALYSIS PER SERVING:
Calories (kcal) 267.69

Protein (g) 7.68	Calories from Protein 30.29	% Calories from Protein 11.32
Carbohydrates(g) 44.27	Calories from Carbohydrates 174.53	% Calories from Carbohydrates 65.20
Fat (g) 7.09	Calories from Fat 62.88	% Calories from Fat 23.49
Saturated Fat (g) 1.12	Total Dietary Fiber (g) 3.99	Sodium (mg) 435.26

CROSTINI WITH ROASTED GARLIC AND GREEN PEA DIP

∞

*T*his dip is a bright spring green and makes a very attractive spread on the toasted crostini. Puréeing the peas helps minimize the insoluble fiber, while the roasted garlic adds a robust taste and tantalizing aroma.

MAKES 4 SERVINGS

> 1 large head garlic, unpeeled
> 1 teaspoon olive oil
> 1 teaspoon white vinegar or white wine vinegar
> ⅛ teaspoon salt
> 3 tablespoons water
> 10-oz. package frozen green peas (about 2 cups),
>   cooked until tender and drained

Two 12" long narrow French bread baguettes, halved horizontally, toasted

Preheat oven to 400°F. Remove outer paper skins from garlic head, but do not separate cloves or peel. Wrap head tightly in foil and bake until soft, about 45 minutes. Cool. Squeeze cloves out of garlic head and into a blender or food processor. Add remaining ingredients and purée until very smooth, scraping down sides with a rubber spatula as necessary. Serve dip with toasted baguettes.

NUTRIENT ANALYSIS PER SERVING:

Calories (kcal) 78.10

Protein (g) 4.26	Calories from Protein 16.45	% Calories from Protein 21.06
Carbohydrates(g) 12.76	Calories from Carbohydrates 49.22	% Calories from Carbohydrates 63.02
Fat (g) 1.43	Calories from Fat 12.43	% Calories from Fat 15.92
Saturated Fat (g) 0.21	Total Dietary Fiber (g) 3.52	Sodium (mg) 153.59

PORTOBELLO MUSHROOM AND SUNDRIED TOMATO BRUSCHETTA

∞

*T*his recipe is a favorite of mine. It's fast, easy, and delicious. It makes a great safe snack in a hurry, and the leftovers are perfect to take to work for lunch the next day.

MAKES 3-4 SERVINGS

½ cup water
¼ cup packed dried tomatoes
1 teaspoon balsamic vinegar
2 portobello mushroom caps, cleaned and chopped (about ¾ lb.)
2 garlic cloves, minced
1 tablespoon olive oil
2 tablespoons finely shredded fresh basil
Salt and pepper to taste

Two 12" long narrow sourdough bread baguettes, halved horizontally, toasted

In a small saucepan heat the water until it boils. Remove from heat and add tomatoes; soak for 15 minutes. Purée tomatoes, cooking water, and vinegar in blender and transfer to serving bowl.

In a medium non-stick skillet sprayed with cooking oil sauté the mushrooms and garlic over medium heat until tender, and the liquid released from mushrooms has evaporated (about 5 minutes). Remove from heat and stir in the olive oil. Fold mushrooms into tomato mixture and add chopped basil. Season with salt and pepper to taste. Serve with baguette.

NUTRIENT ANALYSIS PER SERVING:
Calories (kcal) 253.29

Protein (g) 8.53	Calories from Protein 33.49	% Calories from Protein 13.22
Carbohydrates(g) 42.56	Calories from Carbohydrates 167.14	% Calories from Carbohydrates 65.99
Fat (g) 5.96	Calories from Fat 52.66	% Calories from Fat 20.79
Saturated Fat (g) 0.97	Total Dietary Fiber (g) 3.63	Sodium (mg) 497.47

SMOKED WHITE FISH AND HERB BEAN DIP

∞

*T*his dip not only tastes terrific, it makes a great high-protein, low fat snack. Smoked whitefish is available at most delis.

MAKES 8 SERVINGS

1 15–16 oz. can white beans, rinsed and drained
1 cup smoked whitefish, skinned and boned (about ½ lb.)
Juice from 1 lemon
1 tablespoon olive oil
¼ cup plain rice or soy milk
1 small garlic clove, minced
¼ teaspoon white pepper
1 teaspoon oregano
2 teaspoons basil
1 teaspoon dill weed
Salt and pepper to taste

Four 12" long narrow sourdough baguettes, halved horizontally, toasted

Combine all ingredients in blender and purée until smooth, scraping down sides of blender with a rubber spatula as necessary. Chill and let flavors develop for several hours before serving. Serve with baguette.

NUTRIENT ANALYSIS PER SERVING:
Calories (kcal) 307.14
Protein (g) 17.41
Carbohydrates(g) 48.85
Fat (g) 4.39
Saturated Fat (g) 0.80
Sodium (mg) 727.47

Calories from Protein 70.22
Calories from Carbohydrates 197.09
Calories from Fat 39.83
Cholesterol (mg) 9.74

% Calories from Protein 22.86
% Calories from Carbohydrates 64.17
% Calories from Fat 12.97
Total Dietary Fiber (g) 4.96

SMOKY EGGPLANT HUMMUS

This Lebanese-inspired dip is just plain incredible. The eggplant is the secret to its silky, smoky flavor, and the high soluble fiber of the chickpeas (which are puréed until smooth) make it a safe choice.

MAKES 6-8 SERVINGS

  1 medium eggplant (about 1 pound)
  1 cup cooked or canned chickpeas, rinsed and drained
  1 large garlic clove, mashed
  2 tablespoons well-stirred tahini
  ¼ teaspoon salt
  ¼ cup fresh lemon juice
  1 tablespoon finely chopped fresh flat-leaf parsley

  Pita bread for serving

Preheat broiler or prepare a grill. Prick eggplant in several places with a fork. Broil or grill about 3–4 inches from heat, turning every 10 minutes or so, until eggplant is charred all over and very soft (about 45 minutes). Put eggplant in a bowl to cool and collect juices.

When cold, peel skin off eggplant, discard skin, and transfer pulp to a blender, food processor, or food mill. Add all remaining ingredients except parsley and purée until very smooth, with no visible eggplant seeds, scraping down sides with a rubber spatula as necessary. Transfer to serving bowl and sprinkle with parsley. Serve with fresh pita bread.

NUTRIENT ANALYSIS PER SERVING:
Calories (kcal) 97.95

Protein (g) 4.23	Calories from Protein 15.70	% Calories from Protein 16.03
Carbohydrates(g) 14.81	Calories from Carbohydrates 55.04	% Calories from Carbohydrates 56.19
Fat (g) 3.25	Calories from Fat 27.20	% Calories from Fat 27.77
Saturated Fat (g) 0.44	Total Dietary Fiber (g) 4.52	Sodium (mg) 105.16

GRILLED SHRIMP SHISH KEBABS
WITH SPANISH SAFFRON SAUCE
∞

*B*rilliant golden yellow, smooth and creamy, the pungency of this saffron and garlic sauce plays off the mellow sweetness of grilled shrimp. Shrimp are a great source of protein for an IBS diet because they are so low fat, and the dip is loaded with soluble fiber from the bread and almond base. You won't believe a sauce this rich and creamy could be so safe to eat!

MAKES 6 SERVINGS

1½ pound shrimp, shelled and deveined
1 teaspoon dried rosemary
2 tablespoons olive oil, divided
¼ teaspoon saffron threads
2 cups packed, one-inch cubes of French bread, soaked 15 minutes in ½ cup water
5 large garlic cloves
¼ cup almonds, finely ground
6 tablespoons fresh lemon juice
¼ teaspoon salt
2 tablespoons water

French bread for serving

In a bowl stir together the shrimp, rosemary, and 1 tablespoon olive oil. Chill for 1 hour.

Place saffron threads in a small saucer and microwave for 10–20 seconds, until brittle. Add saffron, remaining 1 tablespoon olive oil, and all other ingredients to a food processor or blender, and purée until smooth, scraping down sides with a rubber spatula as necessary. Transfer dip to serving bowl.

Thread shrimp on metal skewers and grill over medium high heat in grill pan (or over charcoal grill) just until cooked through, about 2 minutes per side. Serve shrimp with saffron sauce and French bread.

NUTRIENT ANALYSIS PER SERVING:
Calories (kcal) 357.55

Protein (g) 29.14	Calories from Protein 117.82	% Calories from Protein 32.95
Carbohydrates(g) 33.33	Calories from Carbohydrates 134.75	% Calories from Carbohydrates 37.69
Fat (g) 11.54	Calories from Fat 104.98	% Calories from Fat 29.36
Saturated Fat (g) 1.73	Cholesterol (mg) 172.37	Total Dietary Fiber (g) 1.92
Sodium (mg) 607.49		

FRESH TEX-MEX GUACAMOLE

*G*uacamole has an undeserved reputation for being high in calories. As you can see from the nutritional analysis, this simply isn't the case. Avocados are high in fat for a fruit—but most fruit contains no fat at all. Guacamole has less than a tablespoon of oil per serving size, and it's full of soluble fiber as well. Served with baked corn chips, guacamole is a perfectly safe, delicious, and very healthy treat. I like the following recipe without the optional seasonings, but feel free to add whatever spices you prefer.

MAKES 3 SERVINGS. RECIPE EASILY DOUBLES.

I large ripe black-skinned California avocado (Hass)
I small clove garlic, mashed to a paste with ¼ teaspoon salt
¼ cup finely diced white onion
I tablespoon fresh lime juice
I tablespoon finely chopped fresh cilantro
Optional seasoning: dash cumin, chili powder, or chipotle powder*

Baked corn chips (Tostitos) for serving

With a fork mash avocado to a smooth paste in serving bowl. Add remaining ingredients, including seasonings if desired, and mix well. Serve with baked corn chips.

*See **Specialty Ingredients** (page 34)

NUTRIENT ANALYSIS PER SERVING:
Calories (kcal) 110.39

Protein (g) 1.49	Calories from Protein 5.47	% Calories from Protein 4.96
Carbohydrates(g) 6.00	Calories from Carbohydrates 22.02	% Calories from Carbohydrates 19.95
Fat (g) 10.03	Calories from Fat 82.90	% Calories from Fat 75.10
Saturated Fat (g) 1.50	Total Dietary Fiber (g) 3.15	Sodium (mg) 8.41

LEMON MARINATED PRAWNS WITH HORSERADISH COCKTAIL SAUCE

This recipe is as versatile as it is scrumptious! It's a terrific picnic standby, an elegant addition to brunch, and a genuine treat to have in the fridge for leftovers. The prawns can be made ahead and kept chilled until you're ready to eat, and if you travel with a small ice chest they make the perfect road food. You won't miss Burger King when you're noshing on these!

MAKES 6 SERVINGS

- 1 lb. shelled and deveined prawns
- 1 tablespoon whole white peppercorns
- 1 tablespoon whole green peppercorns
- 1 bay leaf
- 1½–2 teaspoons ground coriander
- Zest of 1 large lemon
- 3 tablespoons fresh lemon juice
- 3 tablespoons white vinegar
- 2 teaspoons extra-virgin olive oil
- 1 tablespoon water
- 1 tablespoon granulated sugar
- 1 teaspoon salt

Bring a large kettle of water to boil and add prawns, white and green peppercorns, and bay leaf. Cook prawns until just pink and cooked through. Drain. Whisk together remaining ingredients to make marinade. Add shrimp to marinade, tossing to coat. Chill shrimp in marinade, stirring occasionally, at least 8 hours or overnight. Drain shrimp and serve with cocktail sauce.

HORSERADISH COCKTAIL SAUCE:

¼ cup prepared horseradish (nonfat)
¾ cup ketchup
Juice of 1 lemon
Dash Worcestershire sauce
Dash Tabasco sauce (optional)

Combine all ingredients in a small bowl. Makes about 1 cup.

NUTRIENT ANALYSIS PER SERVING:
Calories (kcal) 200.42
Protein (g) 16.89
Carbohydrates(g) 33.82
Fat (g) 2.98
Saturated Fat (g) 0.47
Sodium (mg) 539.41

Calories from Protein 58.94
Calories from Carbohydrates 118.04
Calories from Fat 23.44
Cholesterol (mg) 114.91

% Calories from Protein 29.41
% Calories from Carbohydrates 58.90
% Calories from Fat 11.69
Total Dietary Fiber (g) 1.73

SUMMER TOMATO
AND CILANTRO SALSA
∞

This salsa is a warm weather staple. It perfectly captures the flavors of summer, comes together in a flash, and is terrific with fajitas as well as baked corn chips.

MAKES 4 SERVINGS. RECIPE EASILY DOUBLES.

2 large vine-ripened tomatoes, finely chopped
⅔ cup sweet white onion (such as Walla Walla or Maui), finely chopped
Juice of one lime
6 tablespoons finely chopped fresh cilantro

Baked corn chips (Tostitos) for serving

Combine all ingredients in serving bowl and mix thoroughly. Add more lime juice to taste. Serve with baked corn chips.

NUTRIENT ANALYSIS PER SINGLE SERVING OF SALSA:
Calories (kcal) 32.45

Protein (g) 1.20	Calories from Protein 3.94	% Calories from Protein 12.13
Carbohydrates(g) 7.83	Calories from Carbohydrates 25.67	% Calories from Carbohydrates 79.11
Fat (g) 0.39	Calories from Fat 2.84	% Calories from Fat 8.76
Saturated Fat (g) 0.05	Total Dietary Fiber (g) 1.94	Sodium (mg) 11.43

Sweet Mango and Roasted Tomato Salsa

∞

*P*ositively addictive! I like this salsa smoky, so I add a generous amount of chipotle pepper. I've caught my husband eating this salsa out of the bowl with a spoon. Can't say I blame him.

MAKES 6 SERVINGS

> 5 ripe plum tomatoes
> 1 teaspoon ground chipotle pepper, or to taste*
> ¼ cup fresh lime juice
> 2 tablespoons honey
> 2 small ripe mangoes, peeled and diced
>
> Baked corn chips (Tostitos) for serving

Roast or broil tomatoes until skin blisters and blackens, turning to cook evenly on all sides. Add tomatoes, chipotle, lime, and honey to a blender and purée until smooth. Pour into serving bowl and stir in diced mango. Adjust ratio of lime juice or honey to taste. Serve with baked corn chips.

*See **Specialty Ingredients** (page 34)

NUTRIENT ANALYSIS PER SERVING:
Calories (kcal) 80.45

Protein (g) 0.89	Calories from Protein 3.15	% Calories from Protein 3.91
Carbohydrates (g) 20.96	Calories from Carbohydrates 74.25	% Calories from Carbohydrates 92.30
Fat (g) 0.38	Calories from Fat 3.04	% Calories from Fat 3.78
Saturated Fat (g) 0.07	Total Dietary Fiber (g) 1.93	Sodium (mg) 6.44

TANGY INDIAN TAMARIND CHUTNEY WITH PAPPADAMS

∞

*P*appadams and chutney are like an Indian version of chips and dip. They are a very tasty, low fat snack that will safely satisfy any attack of the munchies.

MAKES 6 SERVINGS

3 tablespoons tamarind concentrate such as TamCon*
¾ cup boiling water
⅔ cup raisins or dates
2 tablespoons granulated sugar
2 teaspoons roasted, ground cumin seeds
4 teaspoons fresh lemon juice
¼ teaspoon cayenne, to taste

Assorted pappadams** (Indian lentil wafers) for serving

Soak the raisins or dates in the boiling water for one hour. Drain. Purée the raisins or dates in a blender with all other ingredients. Will keep in refrigerator for up to 2 months.

Preheat oven broiler. Place pappadams directly on oven racks close to the heat source until bubbled. Watch carefully as they burn quickly. Cool before serving.

*See **Specialty Ingredients** (page 34)

**Pappadams are available in assorted flavors at Indian markets, or see Directory of Resources

NUTRIENT ANALYSIS PER SERVING:
Calories (kcal) 76.48

Protein (g) 0.66	Calories from Protein 2.39	% Calories from Protein 3.12
Carbohydrates (g) 19.79	Calories from Carbohydrates 71.82	% Calories from Carbohydrates 93.91
Fat (g) 0.28	Calories from Fat 2.27	% Calories from Fat 2.97
Saturated Fat (g) 0.05	Total Dietary Fiber (g) 1.39	Sodium (mg) 6.83

HOME-DRIED SWEET AND CHEWY BANANA CHIPS

∞

Home-dried bananas are worlds apart from the nasty store bought deep-fried versions. They are chewy, sweet, and one of the most reliable staples to have on hand for snacking at any time. Not only are they safe and delicious, they're incredibly nutritious. I like to wait for bananas to go on sale and then dry twenty pounds at once. No matter how many batches I make they always disappear too quickly.

SERVINGS VARY

Firm-ripe bananas, in any quantity desired

Peel bananas and gently split horizontally into three segments by inserting index finger at one end until banana naturally segments. Place bananas in a dehydrator or on cookie sheets. Dehydrate according to manufacturer's directions, or in an oven at 200°F for several hours, until dry but still chewy.

NUTRIENT ANALYSIS PER ½ CUP SERVING:
Calories (kcal) 173.00

Protein (g) 1.94	Calories from Protein 6.99	% Calories from Protein 4.04
Carbohydrates(g) 44.14	Calories from Carbohydrates 158.69	% Calories from Carbohydrates 91.73
Fat (g) 0.90	Calories from Fat 7.32	% Calories from Fat 4.23
Saturated Fat (g) 0.35	Total Dietary Fiber (g) 3.75	Sodium (mg) 1.50

CRUNCHY PIZZA PARTY SNACK MIX

This is a wonderful snack food to keep on hand. It's crunchy, spicy, tasty, and everyone loves it. It makes a great party snack alternative to high-fat chips.

MAKES 16 ½ CUP SERVINGS

4 teaspoons dried parsley
½ teaspoon oregano
½ teaspoon basil
½ teaspoon crushed rosemary
1 teaspoon garlic powder
1 teaspoon onion powder
½ teaspoon paprika
1½ teaspoons garlic salt
3 tablespoons fat-free soy blue cheese salad dressing
2 tablespoons tomato paste
2 tablespoons olive oil
⅛ teaspoon liquid smoke*
4 cups Corn Chex cereal
4 cups Rice Chex cereal
2 tablespoons soy Parmesan
1 tablespoon soy Romano

In a small bowl combine first 8 ingredients to form seasoning mix. Set aside. In a very large bowl combine salad dressing, tomato paste, olive oil, and liquid smoke, and blend well. Gradually stir in cereals until evenly coated. Add seasoning mixture. Stir well. Microwave on high for 5–6 minutes, stirring well every 90 seconds, until cooked through. Sprinkle soy Parmesan and soy Romano over cereal mix, stirring well. Cool thoroughly before serving.

*Liquid smoke is a flavoring available in grocery stores in the condiment or spice section. One small bottle will last you a lifetime.

NUTRIENT ANALYSIS PER SERVING:

Calories (kcal) 85.98

Protein (g) 1.42	Calories from Protein 5.76	% Calories from Protein 6.70
Carbohydrates(g) 14.81	Calories from Carbohydrates 59.99	% Calories from Carbohydrates 69.77
Fat (g) 2.22	Calories from Fat 20.23	% Calories from Fat 23.52
Saturated Fat (g) 0.45	Cholesterol (mg) 0.74	Total Dietary Fiber (g) 0.37
Sodium (mg) 386.40		

HONEY GLAZED SNACK MIX

∞

his mix is crunchy, sweet, and salty all at once. I like to make big batches of it and keep bags at work for the afternoon munchies. It's also great snack food for road trips.

MAKES 10 ¹/₂ CUP SERVINGS

3 tablespoons canola oil
¼ cup honey
2 cups Corn Chex cereal
2 cups Rice Chex cereal
I cup mini pretzels

In a small bowl stir together oil and honey until well blended. In a large microwave-safe bowl stir together cereals and pretzels, top with honey mixture, and stir until well combined. Microwave on high for 5–6 minutes, stirring well every 90 seconds, until cooked through. Cool thoroughly before serving.

NUTRIENT ANALYSIS PER SERVING:
Calories (kcal) 206.57

Protein (g) 2.79	Calories from Protein 11.02	% Calories from Protein 5.34
Carbohydrates(g) 35.38	Calories from Carbohydrates 139.81	% Calories from Carbohydrates 67.68
Fat (g) 6.27	Calories from Fat 55.74	% Calories from Fat 26.98
Saturated Fat (g) 0.56	Total Dietary Fiber (g) 0.90	Sodium (mg) 325.09

BREAKFASTS

∞

$\mathcal{B}$ REAKFAST IS THE TRICKIEST meal of the day for IBS, for several reasons. Your stomach is completely empty, and you are probably a little stressed as you're in a hurry to get out the door. You may also be tired because you haven't gotten enough sleep, making your digestion even touchier than usual. The result is that mornings can often trigger problems, and this means that breakfast has to be the safest meal of the day.

For weekday mornings when you don't have much time to cook, here are some fast, safe choices:

Oatmeal made with soymilk, topped with a little brown sugar and sliced banana

Hot cream of rice cereal, topped with maple syrup and diced mango

Toasted plain bagel with a smidgen of soy cream cheese

Toasted sourdough English muffin with marmalade

Toasted French bread with any seedless jam

Toasted French bread with applesauce

Bowl of Rice Chex or Corn Chex with soymilk and a sliced banana

Leftover bowl of Will's Dreamy Lemon Rice Pudding

Leftover bowl of Banana Pecan Breakfast Rice Pudding

Leftover bowl of Indian Pistachio Orange Blossom Tapioca Pudding

Glass of High-Energy Banana Carob Breakfast Shake

Slice of any fruit bread from the Bread Chapter

Have a cup of hot peppermint tea with the above breakfasts and you should be off to a tasty, quick, and safe start to your day.

For more leisurely weekend mornings, or holiday breakfasts and brunches, the recipes in this chapter offer a wide range of delicious, nutritious, and attractive dishes. All of them incorporate cooked fresh fruits or veggies into a high soluble fiber, low fat base.

The really wonderful news here is that although typical breakfast foods such as omelets, pancakes, and French toast are full of triggers like egg yolks, butter, and milk, they are all easily adaptable to the IBS kitchen. By simply using egg whites and no yolks, cooking in non-stick pans without oil, and substituting soy or rice milk for dairy, you can once again enjoy the hearty breakfast treats you love. Who could resist a Mushroom, Crab, and Dill Omelet, a Caramelized Vanilla Pear Pancake, or Cinnamon French Toast with Spiced Plum Sauce, knowing that you don't have to worry about the consequences? I certainly can't—I indulge my morning appetite, and I hope you'll do the same.

HEARTY MEXICAN OMELET
∞

*T*hink you can't eat omelets? Well, you can. The secret is to make them with just egg whites and no yolks, and to cook them without oil in a non-stick frying pan. Feel free to add your favorite seasonings and substitute your favorite veggies.

MAKES 1 SERVING (EASILY DOUBLED OR TRIPLED)

> 2 organic egg whites
> 1/8 teaspoon cumin
> 1/4 teaspoon chili powder
> 1/8 teaspoon garlic salt
> 1 tablespoon diced fresh tomato
> 1 tablespoon diced onion
> 1 tablespoon diced avocado
> 4 large fresh spinach leaves, rinsed and dried, stems removed
> 1 tablespoon finely chopped fresh cilantro

In a small bowl whisk together eggs and spices until lightly frothy. Heat a small non-stick skillet over medium heat, and spray with cooking oil. Add egg mixture and immediately top with diced vegetables, forming a narrow line of filling across the center of the omelet. Add the spinach leaves to cover the vegetable filling, pressing leaves down gently. When edges of the omelet are slightly crisp, carefully fold one side over the filling with a rubber spatula, turn omelet over, and cook on other side for an additional 1–2 minutes. Serve immediately, topped with diced cilantro.

NUTRIENT ANALYSIS PER SERVING:
Calories (kcal) 66.56

Protein (g) 7.74	Calories from Protein 30.58	% Calories from Protein 45.95
Carbohydrates(g) 3.33	Calories from Carbohydrates 13.15	% Calories from Carbohydrates 19.76
Fat (g) 2.57	Calories from Fat 22.82	% Calories from Fat 34.29
Saturated Fat (g) 0.38	Total Dietary Fiber (g) 0.99	Sodium (mg) 421.30

FRESH BASIL OMELET WITH SUNDRIED TOMATOES

∞

This is a fast, delicious, high protein breakfast meal. Serve it with a glass of High-Energy Banana Carob Breakfast Shake (page 40) for a wonderful morning treat in a jiffy.

MAKES 1 SERVING (EASILY DOUBLED OR TRIPLED)

2 organic egg whites
2 tablespoons finely chopped sundried tomatoes
1 tablespoon finely shredded fresh basil
1 tablespoon finely diced onion
1 small garlic clove, mashed

In a small bowl combine egg whites with tomatoes, whisking until lightly frothy. Heat a small non-stick skillet over medium heat, and spray with cooking oil. Add egg mixture and immediately top with remaining ingredients, forming a narrow line of filling across the center of the omelet. When edges of the omelet are slightly crisp, carefully fold one side over the filling with a rubber spatula to completely enclose filling, turn omelet over, and cook on other side for an additional 1–2 minutes. Serve immediately.

NUTRIENT ANALYSIS PER SERVING:
Calories (kcal) 59.80

Protein (g) 8.35	Calories from Protein 32.58	% Calories from Protein 54.49
Carbohydrates(g) 6.42	Calories from Carbohydrates 25.04	% Calories from Carbohydrates 41.88
Fat (g) 0.25	Calories from Fat 2.17	% Calories from Fat 3.63
Saturated Fat (g) 0.04	Total Dietary Fiber (g) 1.18	Sodium (mg) 251.88

MUSHROOM, CRAB, AND DILL OMELET

∞

This is my favorite omelet. I love crab, and the combination of savory sautéed mushrooms with the sweet seafood is irresistible.

MAKES 1 SERVING (EASILY DOUBLED OR TRIPLED)

2 organic egg whites
¼ teaspoon dillweed
⅔ cup finely chopped fresh mushrooms
1 tablespoon finely chopped fresh onion
2 tablespoons crab meat or surimi*

In a small bowl combine egg whites with dill, whisking until lightly frothy. In a small non-stick skillet sprayed with cooking oil, sauté the mushrooms and onions until tender and liquid from mushrooms evaporates. Transfer mushrooms and onions to a small bowl and mix with crab meat. Wipe clean the skillet with a paper towel, spray with cooking oil, and heat over medium. Add egg mixture and immediately top with filling ingredients, forming a narrow line of filling across the center of the omelet. When edges of the omelette are slightly crisp, carefully fold one side over the filling with a rubber spatula to completely enclose filling, turn omelet over, and cook on other side for an additional 1–2 minutes. Serve immediately.

*See **Specialty Ingredients** (page 34)

NUTRIENT ANALYSIS PER SERVING:
Calories (kcal) 63.91

Protein (g) 11.10	Calories from Protein 44.66	% Calories from Protein 69.87
Carbohydrates(g) 3.72	Calories from Carbohydrates 14.97	% Calories from Carbohydrates 23.43
Fat (g) 0.47	Calories from Fat 4.28	% Calories from Fat 6.70
Saturated Fat (g) 0.06	Cholesterol (mg) 14.75	Total Dietary Fiber (g) 0.74
Sodium (mg) 152.87		

HOMEMADE APPLESAUCE

∞

*A*pplesauce is so easy and fast to make you'll wonder why you ever used to buy it. It's a great high soluble snack to have on hand, perfect with toast for breakfast, and a great baking staple that can replace much of the oil in breads and cakes.

MAKES 2 SERVINGS (EASILY DOUBLED)

2 apples, peeled, cored, and chopped

Put the apples in a small saucepan and add just enough water to cover the bottom. Cover and cook over medium low heat, stirring occasionally, until apples disintegrate, about 20 to 30 minutes.

NUTRIENT ANALYSIS PER SERVING:
Calories (kcal) 72.96

Protein (g) 0.19	Calories from Protein 0.70	% Calories from Protein 0.96
Carbohydrates(g) 18.99	Calories from Carbohydrates 69.02	% Calories from Carbohydrates 94.60
Fat (g) 0.40	Calories from Fat 3.25	% Calories from Fat 4.45
Saturated Fat (g) 0.07	Total Dietary Fiber (g) 2.43	

BANANA PECAN BREAKFAST RICE PUDDING
∞

This makes a very flavorful, slightly sweet pudding that is good for breakfasts and snacks.

MAKES 6 SERVINGS

I cup uncooked rose rice
½ teaspoon cinnamon
½ teaspoon nutmeg, freshly ground if possible
½ cup brown sugar
4 cups vanilla soy milk
¼ cup pecans, toasted, finely chopped
2 firm-ripe bananas, diced

Soak rice in cold water for 30 minutes and drain. Rinse and drain again. In a large stockpot add rice and all remaining ingredients except pecans and bananas, stirring well. Bring to a simmer over medium low heat, uncovered, and continue to simmer gently, stirring until rice is tender and begins to disintegrate, about 30 minutes. If pudding becomes too thick add more soy milk as necessary.

Cool pudding and fold in pecans and bananas.

NUTRIENT ANALYSIS PER SERVING:
Calories (kcal) 313.81

Protein (g) 7.76	Calories from Protein 30.03	% Calories from Protein 9.57
Carbohydrates(g) 51.07	Calories from Carbohydrates 197.70	% Calories from Carbohydrates 63.00
Fat (g) 9.88	Calories from Fat 86.08	% Calories from Fat 27.43
Saturated Fat (g) 0.97	Total Dietary Fiber (g) 4.75	Sodium (mg) 26.96

WILL'S DREAMY
LEMON RICE PUDDING

∞

*T*his is unlike any rice pudding you've ever had before. It is a creation of my husband's, and so light and creamy it's practically a mousse. It is the perfect food for IBS, full of soluble fiber and with almost zero fat. It's also delicious any time of day or night. You will not believe something so luscious, smooth, and rich could be such a safe staple. I like to double this recipe and make a big batch on weekends, so I have breakfasts and snacks for the upcoming week.

MAKES 6 SERVINGS

3 cups vanilla soy milk (rice milk will not give as creamy results)
3 cups water
¼ teaspoon salt
½ teaspoon canola oil
¼ cup granulated sugar
5 organic egg whites, whipped until they just barely hold soft peaks
3 cups cold *cooked* short-grain white rice, such as rose, sweet, or sushi rice
Zest of 1 lemon, minced
1 teaspoon vanilla
2 tablespoons chopped raisins (optional)

In a large stockpot,* over medium heat, bring milk and water just barely to a boil. With a metal whisk add in the salt, oil, and sugar. Whisk several large spoonfuls of hot milk into the egg whites to temper them. Add the tempered egg whites to the saucepan of milk and whisk thoroughly, cooking for 2–3 minutes. Add rice and cook, whisking frequently without scraping the bottom of the pan, until mixture thickens slightly, about 20–30 minutes (pudding will thicken further as it cools). Remove from heat and add zest, vanilla, and raisins. Serve warm or chill.

*Because the whipped egg whites in the recipe rise as they cook, it is essential that you use a large stockpot or the pudding will boil over.

NUTRIENT ANALYSIS PER SERVING:
Calories (kcal) 219.99

Protein (g) 8.59	Calories from Protein 34.30	% Calories from Protein 15.59
Carbohydrates(g) 39.94	Calories from Carbohydrates 159.47	% Calories from Carbohydrates 72.49
Fat (g) 2.92	Calories from Fat 26.22	% Calories from Fat 11.92
Saturated Fat (g) 0.34	Total Dietary Fiber (g)* 1.71	Sodium (mg) 157.69

CARAMELIZED VANILLA PEAR PANCAKE

∞

*T*his is a beautiful breakfast dish to serve for holidays or to overnight guests. The pears turn gold-en brown and slightly chewy, and the vanilla perfumes the whole house as the pancake bakes. Everyone with IBS knows that breakfast is the toughest meal, and traditional pancakes are major trig-gers due to their high dairy and fat content. This recipe lets you enjoy a delicious morning treat with-out the fear of consequences.

MAKES 6 SERVINGS

I cup soy or rice milk
I tablespoon apple cider vinegar
1⅓ cups all-purpose unbleached white flour
2 teaspoons baking powder
I teaspoon baking soda
½ teaspoon salt
½ cup brown sugar
4 tablespoons canola oil
8 organic egg whites
2 tablespoons vanilla extract
5 firm-ripe fresh pears
2 tablespoons fresh lemon juice

Preheat oven to 400°F. In a small bowl stir together the soy milk and vinegar; set aside. In a large bowl sift together flour, baking powder, baking soda, salt, and 3 table-spoons of the brown sugar. In a small bowl with an electric mixer beat well 2 table-spoons of the canola oil, soured soy milk, egg whites, and vanilla until frothy. Whisk by hand wet ingredients into dry until just combined. Set batter aside.

Peel and core pears, and slice lengthwise into 8 wedges per pear. Stir together remaining brown sugar and lemon juice, and add pears to coat. In a large cast-iron skil-let heat remaining 2 tablespoons of oil. Arrange pears in a spiral pattern in skillet, top with any remaining sugar mixture, and cook over medium heat until just tender and sugar begins to caramelize, about 10 minutes.

Pour batter over pears and bake in oven for 15 minutes. Reduce oven temperature to 350°F and bake 5–10 minutes more, until golden and firm to touch. Remove from oven, immediately run a thin knife around edge of skillet, place heat-safe plate on top of skillet, and carefully but quickly invert. Slowly lift skillet off cake. Serve immediately.

NUTRIENT ANALYSIS PER SERVING:

Calories (kcal) 384.47

Protein (g) 9.24	Calories from Protein 36.85	% Calories from Protein 9.58
Carbohydrates(g) 62.55	Calories from Carbohydrates 249.45	% Calories from Carbohydrates 64.88
Fat (g) 10.94	Calories from Fat 98.18	% Calories from Fat 25.54
Saturated Fat (g) 0.82	Total Dietary Fiber (g) 4.62	Sodium (mg) 652.16

BANANA CORNMEAL PANCAKES

∞

hese are slightly sweet, richly textured pancakes with the hearty taste of cornmeal. They make a delicious and satisfying breakfast on chilly winter mornings.

MAKES 4-6 SERVINGS

¾ cup soy or rice milk

2 teaspoons apple cider vinegar

2 ripe-black large bananas

½ cup plus 1 tablespoon all-purpose unbleached white flour

1 tablespoon baking powder

2 tablespoons brown sugar

⅓ cup cornmeal

2 organic egg whites

½ teaspoon vanilla

2 tablespoons finely chopped walnuts, lightly toasted (optional)

Pure maple syrup for serving

In a bowl add vinegar to soy milk and stir well. Pour soured milk into blender and add all remaining ingredients (except nuts). Pour batter into bowl or large measuring cup with spout. Heat a non-stick frying pan over medium heat and spray with cooking oil. Pour about ¼ cup of batter at a time onto griddle to form pancakes. Cook until surface bubbles, about 1 minute, and flip pancakes over. Cook until undersides are golden brown and pancakes are cooked through, about 1 minute. Serve immediately with pure maple syrup.

NUTRIENT ANALYSIS PER SERVING:
Calories (kcal) 221.78

Protein (g) 6.51	Calories from Protein 25.25	% Calories from Protein 11.38
Carbohydrates(g) 47.17	Calories from Carbohydrates 182.87	% Calories from Carbohydrates 82.45
Fat (g) 1.57	Calories from Fat 13.66	% Calories from Fat 6.16
Saturated Fat (g) 0.28	Total Dietary Fiber (g) 3.56	Sodium (mg) 402.74

Banana-Banana French Toast with Nutmeg Sugar

∽

*T*his was my favorite French toast growing up. The combination of homemade banana bread with a fresh banana batter simply can't be beat.

MAKES 5 SERVINGS

One loaf homemade Brown Sugar Banana Bread (16 slices) (see recipe, page 98)
2 small bananas, peeled
½ cup vanilla soy milk
5 organic egg whites
1 tablespoon vanilla
Dash nutmeg (freshly grated if possible)

Combine all ingredients except bread in a blender and purée until smooth. Pour batter into 9" pie plate and soak bread slices. Heat a large non-stick skillet over medium high heat and spray with cooking oil. Cook bread slices until lightly golden on each side. Serve sprinkled with nutmeg sugar.

NUTMEG SUGAR:

3 tablespoons sugar
½ teaspoon nutmeg (freshly grated if possible)

Combine nutmeg and sugar in a small bowl and stir well.

NUTRIENT ANALYSIS PER SERVING:
Calories (kcal) 418.06

Protein (g) 9.94	Calories from Protein 10.03	% Calories from Protein 2.40
Carbohydrates(g) 270.40	Calories from Carbohydrates 272.72	% Calories from Carbohydrates 65.24
Fat (g) 15	Calories from Fat 135.30	% Calories from Fat 32.36
Saturated Fat (g) 0.69	Total Dietary Fiber (g) 3.42	Sodium (mg) 411.36

BAKED BLUEBERRY PECAN FRENCH TOAST WITH MAPLE BLUEBERRY SYRUP

∞

Custardy, berry-sweet and with the crunch of toasted pecans, this is a fantastic breakfast dish. It should be prepared the night before so it's ready in a flash the next morning.

MAKES 4 SERVINGS

> One 12" French or sourdough baguette (fresh, not day-old)
> 4 organic egg whites
> 1 cup soy milk
> ¼ teaspoon nutmeg
> 1 teaspoon vanilla
> 4 tablespoons packed brown sugar, divided
> ¼ cup chopped toasted pecans
> ½ cup blueberries, coarsely chopped
> 1 tablespoon canola oil

Spray a 9" square baking dish with cooking oil. Cut 10 one-inch slices from the baguette and arrange in the baking dish. In a large bowl whisk the egg whites until frothy, then whisk in the milk, nutmeg, vanilla, and 2 tablespoons of the brown sugar. Pour evenly over bread, turning slices to coat evenly, cover pan, and chill at least 8 hours or overnight, until liquid is absorbed by bread.

Preheat oven to 400°F. Sprinkle pecans and blueberries evenly over bread. In a small bowl stir together the remaining 2 tablespoons brown sugar and canola oil. Spoon sugar mixture evenly over bread and bake about 20 minutes, until liquid from blueberries is bubbling. Serve with syrup.

Maple Blueberry Syrup

½ cup blueberries
¼ cup pure maple syrup
2 teaspoons fresh lemon juice

In a small saucepan simmer berries and syrup over moderate heat until berries burst, about 5 minutes. Pour syrup through a sieve into a pitcher. Stir in lemon juice.

NUTRIENT ANALYSIS PER SERVING:
Calories (kcal) 316.67

Protein (g) 9.01	Calories from Protein 35.29	% Calories from Protein 11.15
Carbohydrates(g) 53.27	Calories from Carbohydrates 208.58	% Calories from Carbohydrates 65.87
Fat (g) 8.26	Calories from Fat 72.79	% Calories from Fat 22.99
Saturated Fat (g) 0.82	Total Dietary Fiber (g) 3.17	Sodium (mg) 299.81

OLD-FASHIONED VANILLA FRENCH TOAST WITH APRICOT CARAMEL SAUCE

∞

I love French toast, but I went years without being able to eat it because it unfailingly triggered an attack. This version, however, is not only completely safe but absolutely delicious. It's good served with plain old maple syrup, powdered sugar, or fruit jelly, but for a truly decadent treat try the Apricot Caramel Sauce. The toast is slightly crunchy, a little chewy, and the sweet-tart richness of the sauce is the perfect foil.

MAKES 6 SERVINGS

> ½ of a 12.5 oz. package Mori-Nu Silken Lite tofu, drained on a paper towel
> 2 organic egg whites
> ½ cup vanilla soy or rice milk
> 1 tablespoon vanilla
> 1 loaf French baguette or sourdough bread, slightly stale, cut diagonally into 1″ thick slices

Combine first four ingredients in a blender, and blend on high speed until smooth. Pour batter into a glass pie plate. Dip slices of bread in batter, turn over, and soak for about 10 minutes. Heat a large non-stick skillet sprayed with cooking oil over medium high, add bread slices without crowding, and cook until golden brown on the bottom. Turn the slices with a rubber spatula and lightly brown the other sides. Serve immediately with Apricot Caramel Sauce.

NUTRIENT ANALYSIS PER SERVING:
Calories (kcal) 216.04

Protein (g) 9.74	Calories from Protein 40.45	% Calories from Protein 18.72
Carbohydrates(g) 35.68	% Calories from Carbohydrates 68.58	Fat (g) 2.94
Calories from Fat 27.44	% Calories from Fat 12.70	Saturated Fat (g) 0.56
Total Dietary Fiber (g) 2.28	Sodium (mg) 442.36	

APRICOT CARAMEL SAUCE

1½ cups granulated sugar
1 cup water
6–8 fresh ripe apricots, unpeeled, pitted and diced
2 teaspoons vanilla
Juice of half a lemon

In a medium heavy saucepan combine all ingredients except lemon juice and simmer, uncovered, until apricots disintegrate (mash with a potato masher every so often to speed the process) and mixture reduces to a syrup, about 1 hour. Remove from heat and add lemon juice. Makes about 2 cups syrup.

NUTRIENT ANALYSIS PER ¼ CUP SERVING OF SAUCE:
Calories (kcal) 165.78

Protein (g) 0.50	Calories from Protein 1.95	% Calories from Protein 1.18
Carbohydrates(g) 41.74	Calories from Carbohydrates 162.62	% Calories from Carbohydrates 98.09
Fat (g) 0.14	Calories from Fat 1.21	% Calories from Fat 0.73
Saturated Fat (g) 0.01	Total Dietary Fiber (g) 0.85	Sodium (mg) 0.85

CINNAMON FRENCH TOAST WITH SPICED PLUM SAUCE

∞

his French Toast variation is luscious enough to serve to guests. The sauce is cinnamon-sweet and a lovely deep plum hue.

MAKES 6 SERVINGS

½ of a 12.3 oz. package Mori-Nu Silken Lite tofu, drained on a paper towel
2 organic egg whites
½ cup vanilla soy or rice milk
1 teaspoon vanilla
1 teaspoon ground cinnamon
1 loaf French baguette or sourdough bread, slightly stale, cut diagonally into 1" thick slices

Combine first five ingredients in a blender, and blend on high speed until smooth. Pour batter into a glass pie plate. Dip slices of bread in batter, turn over, and soak for about 10 minutes. Heat a large non-stick skillet sprayed with cooking oil over medium high, add bread slices without crowding, and cook until golden brown on the bottom. Turn the slices with a rubber spatula and lightly brown the other sides. Serve immediately with Spiced Plum Sauce.

NUTRIENT ANALYSIS PER SINGLE SERVING OF FRENCH TOAST:
Calories (kcal) 216.04

Protein (g) 9.74	Calories from Protein 40.45	% Calories from Protein 18.72
Carbohydrates(g) 35.68	% Calories from Carbohydrates 68.58	Fat (g) 2.94
Calories from Fat 27.44	% Calories from Fat 12.70	Saturated Fat (g) 0.56
Total Dietary Fiber (g) 2.28	Sodium (mg) 442.36	

Spiced Plum Sauce:

1 cup granulated sugar
1 cup water
6 fresh ripe plums, unpeeled, pitted, and diced
1 cinnamon stick
4 whole cloves
Juice of half a lemon

In a medium heavy saucepan combine all ingredients except lemon juice and simmer, uncovered, until plums completely disintegrate and mixture reduces to a syrup, about 45 minutes. Remove from heat, discard cinnamon stick and cloves, and add lemon juice. Makes about 2 cups syrup.

Nutrient Analysis Per ¼ Cup Serving of Sauce:
Calories (kcal) 127.08

Protein (g) 0.43	Calories from Protein 1.63	% Calories from Protein 1.28
Carbohydrates(g) 32.26	Calories from Carbohydrates 122.31	% Calories from Carbohydrates 96.25
Fat (g) 0.37	Calories from Fat 3.14	% Calories from Fat 2.47
Saturated Fat (g) 0.04	Total Dietary Fiber (g) 1.00	Sodium (mg) 0.99

DECADENT STRAWBERRY—CREAM CHEESE STUFFED FRENCH TOAST WITH FRESH BERRY SYRUP

∞

rench toast doesn't get more extravagantly delicious than this! Make it for Valentine's Day breakfast, Easter brunch, or any other special occasion when you need a morning dish that will knock people's socks off. Or, make a whole batch just for yourself some lazy Sunday morning and revel in it all day long.

MAKES **4** SERVINGS

> 3 oz. soy cream cheese, softened
> ½ cup chopped fresh strawberries
> 1 tablespoon honey
> 16 oz. French bread baguette, sliced diagonally into about 12 pieces
> 4 organic egg whites
> ½ cup vanilla soy milk
> ¼ teaspoon vanilla

In a small bowl beat soy cream cheese until light and fluffy. Add the strawberries and honey, and blend well. Carefully cut a pocket in the center of each bread slice, and fill each pocket with about 1–2 tablespoons of strawberry mixture.

In a medium bowl whisk together egg whites, soy milk, and vanilla, until mixture is slightly frothy. Transfer mixture to shallow pie plate. Soak bread slices in pie plate. Heat a large non-stick skillet over medium heat, and spray with cooking oil. Add bread slices and cook until lightly golden on each side. Serve with warm syrup.

FRESH BERRY SYRUP:

¼ cup fresh chopped blackberries
¼ cup fresh chopped strawberries
½ cup maple syrup

In a small saucepan simmer berries with syrup over medium heat until berries disintegrate and syrup is hot.

NUTRIENT ANALYSIS PER SERVING:
Calories (kcal) 355.71

Protein (g) 16.77	Calories from Protein 67.79	% Calories from Protein 19.06
Carbohydrates(g) 61.97	Calories from Carbohydrates 250.52	% Calories from Carbohydrates 70.43
Fat (g) 4.11	Calories from Fat 37.41	% Calories from Fat 10.52
Saturated Fat (g) 0.93	Cholesterol (mg) 1.70	Total Dietary Fiber (g) 4.01
Sodium (mg) 809.32		

HEAVENLY LEMON FRENCH TOAST WITH BLACKBERRY LEMON SYRUP

∞

This is a simple yet sophisticated French toast that's perfect for sunny summer mornings. French toast is a wonderful breakfast choice for IBS, as the low fat, high soluble fiber foundation allows you to incorporate cooked fresh fruit with minimal risk.

MAKES 6 SERVINGS

½ of a 12.5 oz. package Mori-Nu Silken Lite tofu, drained on a paper towel
2 organic egg whites
½ cup vanilla soy or rice milk
Zest of one large lemon, minced
1 loaf French baguette or sourdough bread, slightly stale, cut diagonally into 1" thick slices

Combine first four ingredients in a blender, and blend on high speed until smooth. Pour batter into a 9" glass pie plate. Dip slices of bread in batter, turn over, and soak for about 10 minutes. Heat a large non-stick skillet sprayed with cooking oil over medium high, add bread slices without crowding, and cook until golden brown on the bottom. Turn the slices with a rubber spatula and lightly brown the other sides. Serve immediately with Blackberry Lemon Syrup.

BLACKBERRY LEMON SYRUP:

½ cup fresh chopped blackberries
½ cup maple syrup
Zest of one large lemon, minced

In a small saucepan simmer all ingredients over medium heat until berries disintegrate and syrup is hot.

NUTRIENT ANALYSIS PER SINGLE SERVING OF FRENCH TOAST:
Calories (kcal) 216.04

Protein (g) 9.74	Calories from Protein 40.45	% Calories from Protein 18.72
Carbohydrates(g) 35.68	% Calories from Carbohydrates 68.58	Fat (g) 2.94
Calories from Fat 27.44	% Calories from Fat 12.70	Saturated Fat (g) 0.56
Total Dietary Fiber (g) 2.28	Sodium (mg) 442.36	

NUTRIENT ANALYSIS PER SERVING OF SYRUP:
Calories (kcal) 75.02

Protein (g) 0.09	Calories from Protein 0.33	% Calories from Protein 0.44
Carbohydrates(g) 19.17	Calories from Carbohydrates 73.82	% Calories from Carbohydrates 98.41
Fat (g) 0.10	Calories from Fat 0.86	% Calories from Fat 1.15
Saturated Fat (g) 0.01	Total Dietary Fiber (g) 0.64	Sodium (mg) 2.36

BLUEBERRY—BROWN SUGAR SCOTTISH OATMEAL

∞

his oatmeal is fast, delicious, nutritious, and ridiculously easy. You simply throw all the ingredients into a bowl and microwave them until the berries burst, creating a swirl of sweet fruit throughout the hearty grain. Cooking the berries makes them much easier to digest, and combining them with the soluble fiber of the oatmeal makes this a safe breakfast choice.

MAKES 1 SERVING*

> ½ cup rolled oatmeal (not instant)
> 1 scant cup vanilla soy or rice milk
> 1 teaspoon brown sugar
> ¼ cup fresh or unthawed frozen whole blueberries

Combine all ingredients in a microwave-safe bowl large enough to prevent boil-over, and stir well. Microwave on high for 2 minutes and stir. Microwave another 1–2 minutes until berries pop and oatmeal is thickened.

*This recipe really needs to be cooked in a microwave, as the stovetop will not give the same results. If you want to make more than one serving, be sure to cook each one in a separate bowl. If you cook a large batch in a single bowl the berries will not burst properly.

NUTRIENT ANALYSIS PER SERVING:
Calories (kcal) 173.43

Protein (g) 9.06	Calories from Protein 33.49	% Calories from Protein 19.31
Carbohydrates(g) 25.97	Calories from Carbohydrates 95.97	% Calories from Carbohydrates 55.34
Fat (g) 5.29	Calories from Fat 43.97	% Calories from Fat 25.35
Saturated Fat (g) 0.63	Total Dietary Fiber (g) 6.36	Sodium (mg) 35.74

BREADS

∽

$\mathcal{B}$READS ARE ONE of the most important staples of the IBS diet. French and sourdough breads are the safest everyday choice, as they are fat-free and low in insoluble fiber. Homemade fruit breads are terrific any time of day or night, for breakfasts, desserts, and snacks, as they combine the goodness of fresh fruit into a low-fat, high soluble fiber base, making them as safe as they are delicious. Breads are easily adaptable to the IBS kitchen. Whole eggs are replaced with egg whites, butter is replaced by canola oil, and fruit purées such as applesauce, pumpkin, or banana substitute for much of the fat while increasing the nutrient value.

Breads are a perfect example of how the special considerations required for IBS cooking do not result in deprivation. You simply haven't had the best banana bread in the world, period, until you've tried my Brown Sugar Banana Bread. There's no flavor missing, just fat. It's equally impossible to feel deprived when you're snacking on a warm piece of Sweet Cinnamon Zucchini Bread, Pumpkin Apple Spice Bread, or my grandmother's heirloom Chocolate Applesauce Cake. So get in the habit of baking large batches of bread every other weekend or so, freeze the extra loaves, and you'll always have a delicious, healthy, and safe staple on hand for yourself as well as a special treat for the rest of your family to enjoy.

BROWN SUGAR BANANA BREAD

This bread is a slight variation of my grandmother's recipe. I was raised by my grandparents and I learned to cook at the side of my beloved Grams. Just the smell of this bread baking takes me instantly back to my childhood and those rainy afternoons whiled away in the warmth and comfort of the kitchen. This recipe is, without a doubt, the best banana bread in the world, and it makes absolutely spectacular French toast as well (see page 85).

MAKES TWO 9 X 5" LOAVES, 16 SLICES PER LOAF

Preheat oven to 350°F.
Sift into a large bowl:
   3½ cups all-purpose unbleached white flour
   ½ teaspoon baking powder
   2 teaspoons baking soda
   ½ teaspoon salt

Whisk dry ingredients with a wire whisk or fork until well blended.

In a large bowl blend with an electric mixer until creamy:
   6 organic egg whites
   ⅓ cup canola oil
   1⅓ cup brown sugar
   1 tablespoon vanilla
   3 cups mashed black bananas (6–8 bananas)*

Add dry ingredients to wet and with a few swift strokes of a wooden spoon blend by hand until smooth. Pour into non-stick loaf pans sprayed with cooking oil and bake for 50–60 minutes or until a toothpick or cake tester inserted into the center of the loaf comes out clean. Cool on rack. Recipe doubles or triples easily, and extra loaves freeze well.

*The bananas have to be super-ripe for this recipe. If they're not black, they're not ready.

NUTRIENT ANALYSIS PER SLICE:
Calories (kcal) 126.88

Protein (g) 2.29	Calories from Protein 8.99	% Calories from Protein 7.08
Carbohydrates (g) 24.38	Calories from Carbohydrates 95.75	% Calories from Carbohydrates 75.46
Fat (g) 2.51	Calories from Fat 22.15	% Calories from Fat 17.45
Saturated Fat (g) 0.22	Total Dietary Fiber (g) 0.88	Sodium (mg) 136.94

SWEET-TART
ORANGE CRANBERRY BREAD
∞

his bread is wonderful toasted and served as a snack with a nice hot cup of tea. For an easy variation, substitute currants for the cranberries.

MAKES ONE 9 X 5" LOAF, 16 SLICES PER LOAF

3 cups all-purpose unbleached white flour
1 tablespoon baking powder
½ teaspoon salt
¾ cup granulated sugar
2 tablespoons cornstarch
1 cup vanilla soy milk
1 tablespoon apple cider vinegar
2 tablespoons orange zest (from about 2 oranges)
½ cup fresh orange juice
¼ cup canola oil
1 cup chopped fresh or dried cranberries

Preheat oven to 350°F. In a large bowl sift together dry ingredients, and stir well with a wire whisk or fork to thoroughly blend. Set aside. In a small bowl combine vinegar and soy milk and set aside. In a medium bowl whisk together orange juice, zest, oil, and vinegar/soy milk mixture. Blend well. Stir cranberries into wet ingredients. Add wet ingredients to dry with a few swift strokes of a wooden spoon just until blended. Pour into non-stick loaf pan sprayed with cooking oil; smooth batter evenly with a rubber spatula. Bake for about 1 hour or until a toothpick or cake tester inserted into the center of the loaf comes out clean. Cool on rack.

NUTRIENT ANALYSIS PER SLICE:
Calories (kcal) 168.38

Protein (g) 2.92	Calories from Protein 11.62	% Calories from Protein 6.90
Carbohydrates(g) 30.29	Calories from Carbohydrates 120.51	% Calories from Carbohydrates 71.57
Fat (g) 4.05	Calories from Fat 36.25	% Calories from Fat 21.53
Saturated Fat (g) 0.32	Total Dietary Fiber (g) 1.11	Sodium (mg) 166.73

OLD-FASHIONED
ORANGE BLOSSOM BREAD

∞

*T*his is a wonderful bread that is rich with essence of fresh oranges and the subtle, unusual note of orange flower water as well. It is sweet, sticky, and a safe indulgence for breakfast or an afternoon snack.

MAKES ONE 9 x 5" LOAF, 16 SLICES PER LOAF

    ¾ cup soy or rice milk
    2 teaspoons apple cider vinegar
    2 cups all-purpose unbleached white flour
    1½ teaspoons baking powder
    ½ teaspoon salt
    1½ cups granulated sugar
    ¼ cup plus 2 tablespoons canola oil
    4 organic egg whites
    Zest from 2 oranges
    1 teaspoon orange flower water*

Preheat oven to 350°F. In a medium bowl add vinegar to soy milk and stir well; set aside. Sift dry ingredients into large bowl. Whisk well to combine. Add to vinegar/soy milk mixture the oil, egg whites, zest, and orange flower water. Whisk well until thoroughly combined. Add wet ingredients to dry with a few swift strokes of a wooden spoon just until blended. Pour batter into a non-stick loaf pan sprayed with cooking oil. Bake for about 1 hour or until a toothpick or cake tester inserted into the center of the loaf comes out clean.

GLAZE:

Strained juice from 1 orange
1 tablespoon granulated sugar
1 teaspoon orange flower water*

While bread is baking, stir glaze ingredients together until sugar dissolves. When bread is done, and while it is still hot from the oven, run a knife around the edges of the pan to loosen the loaves, and prick bread carefully all over with a thin wooden or metal skewer. Pour glaze over bread, and cool in pans on rack.

*See **Specialty Ingredients** (page 34)

NUTRIENT ANALYSIS PER SLICE:
Calories (kcal) 188.34

Protein (g) 2.85	Calories from Protein 11.25	% Calories from Protein 5.97
Carbohydrates(g) 32.45	Calories from Carbohydrates 128.25 %	Calories from Carbohydrates 68.09
Fat (g) 5.49	Calories from Fat 48.84	% Calories from Fat 25.93
Saturated Fat (g) 0.41	Total Dietary Fiber (g) 0.58	Sodium (mg) 134.02

SWEET CINNAMON ZUCCHINI BREAD
∞

*T*his is another one of my grandmother's delicious old-fashioned recipes. It's just slightly sweet, very moist, and so heavenly it's hard to believe it's good for you. The zucchini makes for a wonderfully moist texture with very little oil, and provides lots of nutrients as well.

MAKES TWO SMALL 9 X 5" LOAVES, 12 SLICES PER LOAF
IF THE RECIPE IS DOUBLED IT WILL MAKE TWO FULL-SIZE 9 X5" LOAVES,
12 SLICES PER LOAF

Preheat oven to 325°F.
Sift into a large bowl:

3 cups all-purpose unbleached white flour
1 teaspoon salt
1 teaspoon soda
1 tablespoon cinnamon
¼ teaspoon baking powder

Whisk dry ingredients with a wire whisk or fork until thoroughly blended.
In a large bowl beat well with an electric mixer:

6 organic egg whites, beaten light and foamy
½ cup canola oil
1½ cups brown sugar
2 cups grated unpeeled zucchini
2 teaspoons vanilla

Add dry ingredients to wet with a few swift strokes of a wooden spoon just until blended. Pour batter into two non-stick loaf pans sprayed with cooking oil. Bake for about 1 hour or until a toothpick or cake tester inserted into the center of the loaf comes out clean. Cool on racks.

NUTRIENT ANALYSIS PER SLICE:
Calories (kcal) 138.49

Protein (g) 2.62	Calories from Protein 10.49	% Calories from Protein 7.57
Carbohydrates(g) 21.41	Calories from Carbohydrates 85.57	% Calories from Carbohydrates 61.79
Fat (g) 4.72	Calories from Fat 42.43	% Calories from Fat 30.64
Saturated Fat (g) 0.35	Total Dietary Fiber (g) 0.70	Sodium (mg) 172.37

CINNAMON LIME PECAN BREAD
∞

*T*his is an unusual, subtly flavored bread with the scent of fresh limes. It's delicious toasted.

MAKES ONE 9 X 5" LOAF, 16 SLICES PER LOAF

3 cups all-purpose unbleached white flour
1 tablespoon baking powder
½ teaspoon salt
½ teaspoon cinnamon
1 cup granulated sugar
2 tablespoons cornstarch
1 cup vanilla soy milk
1 tablespoon apple cider vinegar
2 tablespoons lime zest (from about 4 limes)
½ cup fresh lime juice
¼ cup canola oil
⅓ cup chopped pecans

Preheat oven to 350°F. In a large bowl sift together dry ingredients, and stir well with a wire whisk or fork to thoroughly blend. Set aside. In a small bowl combine vinegar and soy milk and set aside. In a medium bowl whisk together lime juice, zest, oil, and vinegar/soy milk mixture. Blend well. Stir pecans into wet ingredients. Add wet ingredients to dry with a few swift strokes of a wooden spoon just until blended. Pour into non-stick loaf pan sprayed with cooking oil; smooth batter evenly with a rubber spatula. Bake for about 1 hour or until a toothpick or cake tester inserted into the center of the loaf comes out clean. Cool on rack.

NUTRIENT ANALYSIS PER SLICE:
Calories (kcal) 191.86

Protein (g) 3.07	Calories from Protein 12.10	% Calories from Protein 6.31
Carbohydrates(g) 33.00	Calories from Carbohydrates 130.01	% Calories from Carbohydrates 67.76
Fat (g) 5.61	Calories from Fat 49.76	% Calories from Fat 25.93
Saturated Fat (g) 0.45	Total Dietary Fiber (g) 1.06	Sodium (mg) 166.73

SUNSHINE BREAD

∞

This bread is a beautiful brilliant orange and guaranteed to make any morning a little sunnier. Lusciously moist and heady with spices, it is also a delicious way to incorporate sweet potatoes, one of the most nutritious and high-soluble fiber vegetables, into your diet.

MAKES TWO 9 x 5" LOAVES, 16 SLICES PER LOAF

Preheat oven to 350°F.

In a large bowl sift:

3½ cups all-purpose unbleached white flour

2 teaspoons baking soda

½ teaspoon baking powder

½ teaspoon salt

2 teaspoons cinnamon

1 teaspoon cloves

Whisk dry ingredients with a wire whisk or fork until thoroughly blended.

In a small bowl stir together and set aside:

⅔ cup soy or rice milk

2 teaspoons apple cider vinegar

In a large bowl beat well with an electric mixer:

2⅔ cups brown sugar

⅔ cup canola oil

8 organic egg whites

4 cups finely diced sweet potatoes, steamed until very soft, then puréed until
    smooth

2 tablespoons vanilla

Beat in the vinegar/soy milk mixture. With a wooden spoon, add the dry ingredients to the wet, stirring the batter by hand just until well blended. Fold in by hand:

½ cup finely chopped raisins
½ cup finely chopped dates

Pour batter into two non-stick loaf pans sprayed with cooking oil. Bake for about 1 hour or until a toothpick or cake tester inserted into the center of the loaf comes out clean. Cool on racks.

NUTRIENT ANALYSIS PER SLICE:
Calories (kcal) 169.04

Protein (g) 2.91	Calories from Protein 11.45	% Calories from Protein 6.77
Carbohydrates(g) 28.96	Calories from Carbohydrates 114.14	% Calories from Carbohydrates 67.52
Fat (g) 4.90	Calories from Fat 43.45	% Calories from Fat 25.70
Saturated Fat (g) 0.41	Total Dietary Fiber (g) 1.72	Sodium (mg) 144.06

LEMON-GLAZED STICKY BREAD
∞

*O*oh, this bread is tart, sweet, and sticky-rich. It is intensely lemony and will perfume your whole house as it bakes. Don't forget the glaze—the bread just isn't the same without it. If you can stand to, let this bread sit for a day—it's better the day after it's baked.

MAKES ONE 9 x 5" LOAF, 16 SLICES PER LOAF

¾ cup soy or rice milk
2 teaspoons apple cider vinegar
2 cups all-purpose unbleached white flour
1½ teaspoons baking powder
½ teaspoon salt
1½ cups granulated sugar
¼ cup plus 2 tablespoons canola oil
4 organic egg whites
Zest from 2 lemons, minced

GLAZE:

Strained juice from 2 lemons
3 tablespoons granulated sugar

Preheat oven to 350°F. In a medium bowl add vinegar to soy milk and stir well; set aside. Sift dry ingredients into large bowl. Whisk well to combine. Add to vinegar/soy milk mixture the oil, egg whites, and zest. Whisk well until thoroughly combined. Add wet ingredients to dry with a few swift strokes of a wooden spoon just until blended. Pour batter into a non-stick loaf pan sprayed with cooking oil. Bake for about 1 hour or until a toothpick or cake tester inserted into the center of the loaf comes out clean.

While bread is baking, stir glaze ingredients together until sugar dissolves. When bread is done, and while it is still hot from the oven, run a knife around the edges of the pan to loosen the loaves, and prick bread carefully all over with a thin wooden or metal skewer. Pour glaze over bread, and cool in pan on rack.

NUTRIENT ANALYSIS PER SLICE:
Calories (kcal) 189.98

Protein (g) 2.83	Calories from Protein 11.14	% Calories from Protein 5.86
Carbohydrates(g) 33.02	Calories from Carbohydrates 130.21	% Calories from Carbohydrates 68.54
Fat (g) 5.48	Calories from Fat 48.63	% Calories from Fat 25.60
Saturated Fat (g) 0.41	Total Dietary Fiber (g) 0.59	Sodium (mg) 134.02

PUMPKIN APPLE SPICE BREAD

*E*verybody's favorite bread. This is moist, richly spiced, and just plain wonderful.

MAKES TWO 9 x 5" LOAVES, 16 SLICES PER LOAF

Preheat oven to 350°F.

TOPPING:

- 1 tablespoon all-purpose unbleached white flour
- 5 tablespoons brown sugar
- 1 teaspoon cinnamon
- 1 tablespoon canola oil

Combine all ingredients in a small bowl. Set aside.

Sift into a large bowl:
- 3 cups all-purpose unbleached white flour
- ¾ teaspoon salt
- 2 teaspoons baking soda
- 1½ teaspoons cinnamon
- 1 teaspoon nutmeg
- 1 teaspoon cloves
- ¼ teaspoon allspice
- ¼ teaspoon ginger

Whisk dry ingredients with a wire whisk or fork until thoroughly blended.

In a large bowl beat well with an electric mixer:
  16 oz. can pumpkin
  ¾ cup canola oil
  2¼ cups granulated sugar
  8 organic egg whites

Fold into wet ingredients:
  2 large Granny Smith apples, peeled and chopped (about 2 cups)

With a wooden spoon, add the dry ingredients to the wet, stirring the batter by hand until well blended. Pour batter into two non-stick loaf pans sprayed with cooking oil. Sprinkle on topping. Bake for about 50 minutes or until a toothpick or cake tester inserted into the center of the loaf comes out clean. Cool on racks.

NUTRIENT ANALYSIS PER SLICE:
Calories (kcal) 166.39

Protein (g) 2.28	Calories from Protein 8.98	% Calories from Protein 5.40
Carbohydrates(g) 27.10	Calories from Carbohydrates 106.68	% Calories from Carbohydrates 64.11
Fat (g) 5.73	Calories from Fat 50.73	% Calories from Fat 30.49
Saturated Fat (g) 0.44	Total Dietary Fiber (g) 0.89	Sodium (mg) 148.50

MY GREAT-GREAT-GRANDMOTHER'S CHOCOLATE APPLESAUCE CAKE

∞

*M*y grandmother learned this recipe from her mother, who in turn had learned it from hers. I grew up watching my Grams bake this cake frequently, and it is now one of my own most cherished standbys. I still follow the directions from the original recipe card written in my grandmother's lovely old-fashioned handwriting, although I have made several adaptations. I replaced the butter with canola oil, and I reduced the amount of oil by increasing the applesauce. Although this is called a cake, it is baked in bread loaf pans and is not really dessert-sweet—it is better suited to breakfasts. Easy enough for children to bake, the cake comes out perfectly every time, and it is dependably scrumptious. I consider this my most treasured recipe.

MAKES TWO 9 X 5" LOAVES, 16 SLICES PER LOAF

Preheat oven to 325°F.
Sift together in large bowl and stir thoroughly to combine:
   4 cups all-purpose unbleached white flour
   4 teaspoons baking soda
   ½ cup unsweetened cocoa powder
   2 tablespoons cornstarch
   2 cups granulated sugar
   1 teaspoon cinnamon
   1 teaspoon cloves
   1 teaspoon nutmeg
   1 teaspoon salt

Whisk together by hand thoroughly:
   3½ cups homemade or unsweetened bottled applesauce
   ½ cup canola oil
   2 tablespoons vanilla
   2 cups diced raisins

Add the wet ingredients to the dry with a few swift strokes of a wooden spoon until well blended. Pour batter into two non-stick loaf pans sprayed with cooking oil. Bake for 1 hour to 1 hour 15 minutes, or until a toothpick or cake tester inserted into the center of the loaf comes out clean. Cool on racks.

NUTRIENT ANALYSIS PER SLICE:
Calories (kcal) 182.11

Protein (g) 2.23	Calories from Protein 8.65	% Calories from Protein 4.75
Carbohydrates(g) 36.02	Calories from Carbohydrates 139.90	% Calories from Carbohydrates 76.82
Fat (g) 3.84	Calories from Fat 33.56	% Calories from Fat 18.43
Saturated Fat (g) 0.41	Total Dietary Fiber (g) 1.63	Sodium (mg) 232.64

GINGERBREAD

∽

*G*ingerbread is one of my childhood favorites, and I hope this delectably spicy recipe becomes one of yours. Ginger is very soothing to the GI tract, and this rich, moist bread is low fat as well. Enjoy without worry!

MAKES 8 SERVINGS

Preheat oven to 350°F. Spray a 9" square baking pan with cooking oil and set aside. Sift together in a large bowl:

1½ cups all-purpose unbleached white flour
½ cup brown sugar
1¼ teaspoons baking soda
1 teaspoon cinnamon
2 teaspoons ground ginger
½ teaspoon cloves
½ teaspoon nutmeg
⅛ teaspoon salt

Whisk dry ingredients with a wire whisk or fork until thoroughly blended.

In a medium bowl beat together:

½ cup molasses
½ cup fresh orange juice, strained
4 organic egg whites
3 tablespoons canola oil
1½ tablespoons finely grated fresh gingerroot
2 tablespoons finely chopped crystallized ginger
2 teaspoons vanilla

Add the wet ingredients to the dry with a few swift strokes of a wooden spoon. Pour batter into prepared pan and bake for 35–40 minutes, or until a toothpick or cake tester inserted into the center of the gingerbread comes out clean. Cool on rack.

NUTRIENT ANALYSIS PER SLICE:
Calories (kcal) 233.10

Protein (g) 4.31	Calories from Protein 17.32	% Calories from Protein 7.43
Carbohydrates(g) 41.25	Calories from Carbohydrates 165.85	% Calories from Carbohydrates 71.15
Fat (g) 5.52	Calories from Fat 49.93	% Calories from Fat 21.42
Saturated Fat (g) 0.42	Total Dietary Fiber (g) 0.69	Sodium (mg) 276.05

SIMPLE SWEET CORNBREAD
∞

lthough traditional Southern corn bread is baked in a cast-iron skillet for a crunchy texture, this recipe uses a non-stick loaf pan in order to reduce the fat content. The moist interior and sweet corn goodness remain.

MAKES ONE 9 X 5" LOAF, 16 SLICES PER LOAF

Preheat oven to 350°F.

1½ cups soy milk
1½ tablespoons apple cider vinegar
1 cup yellow cornmeal
1 cup all-purpose unbleached white flour
½ cup granulated sugar
½ teaspoon salt
1 teaspoon baking powder
½ teaspoon baking soda
¼ cup canola oil
1 organic egg white

In a medium bowl stir together the soy milk and vinegar; set aside. Sift into a large bowl the cornmeal, flour, sugar, salt, baking powder, and baking soda. Stir together with a wire whisk until well combined. Set aside. To the vinegar/soy milk mixture add the oil and egg whites. Mix well with a wire whisk until thoroughly combined. Add the wet ingredients to the dry with a few swift strokes of a wooden spoon. Pour batter into a non-stick loaf pan sprayed with cooking oil. Bake for 40–45 minutes, or until a toothpick or cake tester inserted into the center of the loaf comes out clean. Cool on a rack.

NUTRIENT ANALYSIS PER SLICE:
Calories (kcal) 123.28

Protein (g) 2.39	Calories from Protein 9.49	% Calories from Protein 7.70
Carbohydrates(g) 19.51	Calories from Carbohydrates 77.47	% Calories from Carbohydrates 62.84
Fat (g) 4.06	Calories from Fat 36.32	% Calories from Fat 29.46
Saturated Fat (g) 0.32	Total Dietary Fiber (g) 1.15	Sodium (mg) 149.15

GARLIC ROSEMARY FRENCH BREAD
∞

*lthough this recipe takes some time, the result is simply fabulous. Spend a rainy afternoon bak-
ing and this bread will be your just reward. It is wonderful warm from the oven or toasted.*

MAKES 2 LOAVES, 16 SLICES PER LOAF

BREAD:

2¾–3¾ cups all-purpose unbleached white flour
1 tablespoon granulated sugar
2 teaspoons garlic salt*
2 teaspoons garlic powder*
2 teaspoons onion powder*
1 teaspoon crushed rosemary
2 packages active dry yeast
2 tablespoons olive oil
2 cups all-purpose unbleached white flour
1 tablespoon water
1 organic egg white

FILLING:

2 tablespoons soy Parmesan
2 tablespoons dried minced onion*
1½ teaspoons garlic powder*
1 teaspoon crushed rosemary
1 large garlic clove, minced
¼ cup minced onion
2 tablespoons olive oil, divided

In a large bowl combine 2 cups flour, sugar, salt, seasonings, and yeast; blend well
with a wooden spoon. In a small saucepan or the microwave heat 2 cups water and oil
until 120–130°F. Add liquid to flour mixture, blend with an electric mixer at low speed
until moistened, then blend 3 minutes more at medium speed. With a wooden spoon

stir in 2 cups flour, then an additional ½–1 cup flour until dough pulls cleanly away from sides of bowl. On a floured surface knead in ¼–¾ cup flour until dough is smooth and elastic, about five minutes.

Place dough in a lightly greased bowl; cover with plastic wrap and a towel. Let rise in a warm, draft-free place (about 75–85°F) for about 45 minutes or until doubled in size. Punch down dough, cut in half, and shape in to balls. Roll out each ball into a 12 x 8" rectangle. Brush each rectangle with 1 tablespoon olive oil. Mix remaining filling ingredients in a small bowl and sprinkle evenly over each rectangle. Roll up each rectangle from the long side, pinwheel style. Pinch ends and seam tightly closed; place seam-side down on a cookie sheet sprayed with cooking oil. Cover loaves with plastic wrap and towels, place in a warm draft-free place, and let rise about 10–15 minutes or until doubled in size.

Preheat oven to 375°F. Blend 1 tablespoon of water with the egg white, and brush lightly over each loaf. Sprinkle loaves with garlic salt. Bake 30–40 minutes, until golden brown. Cool on wire racks.

*Do not substitute fresh herbs or spices for the dried versions in this recipe, as the results will not be the same.

NUTRIENT ANALYSIS PER SLICE:
Calories (kcal) 102.05

Protein (g) 2.75	Calories from Protein 11.14	% Calories from Protein 10.92
Carbohydrates(g) 17.86	Calories from Carbohydrates 72.44	% Calories from Carbohydrates 70.98
Fat (g) 2.02	Calories from Fat 18.47	% Calories from Fat 18.10
Saturated Fat (g) 0.33	Cholesterol (mg) 0.25	Total Dietary Fiber (g) 0.72
Sodium (mg) 153.60		

PARISIAN BAGUETTE

∞

*T*his is an easy, delicious recipe for one of the IBS kitchen staples. If you can't get good fresh French bread in your area, consider baking your own. The result is well-worth the effort.

MAKES 1 BAGUETTE, ABOUT 16 SLICES (RECIPE DOUBLES EASILY)

1 teaspoon active dry yeast
1 teaspoon granulated sugar
1½ cups lukewarm water
4–4½ cups all-purpose unbleached white flour
2 teaspoons salt

In a large bowl, sprinkle yeast and sugar over warm water (about 100–115°F) and let sit until foamy, about 4–5 minutes. Stir in 2 cups flour until combined. Add salt and another 2 cups flour and stir until mixture forms a stiff dough.

On a lightly floured surface knead dough until smooth and elastic, about 8–10 minutes, gradually kneading in remaining ½ cup flour as needed if dough is sticky. Place dough in a lightly oiled large bowl, cover bowl with plastic wrap and a kitchen towel, and let rise in a warm draft-free spot (about 75-85°F) until doubled, about 1½ hours.

Preheat oven to 400°F. Punch down dough and form into a long narrow baguette, roughly 20 inches by 3 inches. Place loaf diagonally on a lightly greased cookie sheet and let rise, uncovered, in a warm draft-free spot, about 30 minutes.

Make 3 diagonal slashes on top of loaf with a small sharp knife, and lightly mist top of loaf with water. Bake loaf in center of oven until golden, about 30 minutes, and cool on a rack.

NUTRIENT ANALYSIS PER SLICE:
Calories (kcal) 129.72

Protein (g) 3.73	Calories from Protein 15.25	% Calories from Protein 11.75
Carbohydrates(g) 27.19	Calories from Carbohydrates 111.20	% Calories from Carbohydrates 85.72
Fat (g) 0.36	Calories from Fat 3.28	% Calories from Fat 2.53
Saturated Fat (g) 0.06	Total Dietary Fiber (g) 1.00	Sodium (mg) 291.52

SIDE DISHES
AND SALADS

∽

SIDE DISHES AND SALADS offer a great opportunity to add more soluble fiber to your meals, and it's quite easy to do so deliciously. Potatoes, probably the most traditional American side dish, are a terrific staple for the IBS kitchen and can be cooked an infinite variety of safe and tasty ways. Favorite family recipes such as scalloped potatoes can be easily adapted with soy or rice milk, and standbys like crispy hash browns can be cooked in a non-stick skillet for plenty of crunch without the oil. Think of sweet potatoes when you want a change of pace as they're absolutely crammed with nutrients. Traditional green salads, a trigger food due to their high insoluble fiber content and typically oil-based dressings, are best eaten in small quantities and only at the end of meals, never on an empty stomach. For salads that can be safely eaten as meals in their own right, try delicious alternatives like Italian Tuna, Lemon and Basil Pasta Salad, Roasted Sweet Potato Cider Salad, or Tangy Thai Salad with Fresh Herbs.

CRUNCHY SKILLET-BROWNED GARLIC NEW POTATOES

∞

*S*uper easy and outrageously delicious, these potatoes are crispy-crunchy outside, creamy smooth inside, and have an addictive garlicky twist. Serve as a dinner side dish or as breakfast home-fries to die for. Don't worry about leftovers—I promise you there won't be any. And don't worry about an attack—this dish is almost pure soluble fiber.

A non-stick pan is essential to the success of this recipe.

MAKES 4 SERVINGS

2 lbs. small red or white new potatoes, scrubbed, peeled, and quartered
1 tablespoon olive oil
6 large garlic cloves, minced
1 teaspoon garlic salt

Place potatoes in a large, non-stick skillet. Add cold water to cover the potatoes by three-fourths. Add the oil, garlic, and salt. Bring to a boil, reduce heat to medium, and cook until water evaporates, turning potatoes occasionally, about 25 minutes. Increase heat to medium-high and cook until potatoes are crispy and brown, turning frequently, about 10–15 minutes. Serve immediately.

NUTRIENT ANALYSIS PER SERVING:
Calories (kcal) 215.71

Protein (g) 4.98	Calories from Protein 19.39	% Calories from Protein 8.99
Carbohydrates (g) 42.27	Calories from Carbohydrates 164.57	% Calories from Carbohydrates 76.29
Fat (g) 3.62	Calories from Fat 31.75	% Calories from Fat 14.72
Saturated Fat (g) 0.52	Total Dietary Fiber (g) 3.72	Sodium (mg) 297.5

CANDIED SWEET POTATOES
∞

O h, I love these candied sweet potatoes! They are rich and tender with a chewy caramelized crust. Their luscious sweetness is offset by just a hint of spiciness from the cayenne. This recipe makes my favorite Thanksgiving side dish.

MAKES 6 SERVINGS

> 2 tablespoons canola oil
> 3 large sweet potatoes, peeled and cut into ¼″ slices
> 1 cup water
> ½ cup packed brown sugar
> Dash salt
> Dash cayenne, or to taste

Heat the oil in a well-seasoned large cast iron skillet over medium low heat. Add the sweet potatoes. Stir together the water, sugar, salt, and cayenne, and pour over potatoes. Cover and cook for about 20 minutes without stirring. Turn the potatoes over, cover, and cook for about 15 minutes more, turning occasionally to coat each piece with syrup and taking care that the potatoes caramelize evenly. Continue to cook and turn potatoes in this manner until they are fork-tender. Transfer to serving platter immediately.

NUTRIENT ANALYSIS PER SERVING:
Calories (kcal) 178.44

Protein (g) 1.07	Calories from Protein 4.19	% Calories from Protein 2.35
Carbohydrates(g) 33.62	Calories from Carbohydrates 131.47	% Calories from Carbohydrates 73.68
Fat (g) 4.86	Calories from Fat 42.77	% Calories from Fat 23.97
Saturated Fat (g) 0.37	Total Dietary Fiber (g) 1.95	Sodium (mg) 41.44

KOREAN SEASONED POTATOES

∽

*T*hese potatoes are a type of panchan, the little side dishes served with rice at every Korean meal. They are rather unusual and very tasty. Drizzle any extra marinade on cooked fish, steamed green vegetables, and rose rice, then add the potatoes, and you'll have a wonderful and healthy meal in minutes.

MAKES 4 SERVINGS

> 2 large russet potatoes
> 2 tablespoons Japanese soy sauce such as Kikkoman
> 2 teaspoons brown sugar
> 1 tablespoon minced garlic (about 2 medium cloves)
> 1 tablespoon toasted sesame seeds (crush slightly with a mortar and pestle or in a spice grinder)*
> 2 teaspoons toasted sesame oil*

Peel potatoes and cut into 1″ matchsticks. Place in large saucepan with enough cold water to barely cover. Bring to a boil and cook until just fork-tender, about 3–4 minutes. Do not overcook. Drain.

In serving bowl mix remaining ingredients well. Add drained potatoes and toss to coat. Chill thoroughly for 1–2 hours before serving.

*See **Specialty Ingredients** (page 34)

NUTRIENT ANALYSIS PER SERVING:
Calories (kcal) 118.23

Protein (g) 3.32	Calories from Protein 12.86	% Calories from Protein 10.88
Carbohydrates(g) 19.72	Calories from Carbohydrates 76.30	% Calories from Carbohydrates 64.54
Fat (g) 3.34	Calories from Fat 29.06	% Calories from Fat 24.58
Saturated Fat (g) 0.48	Total Dietary Fiber (g) 1.93	Sodium (mg) 509.98

STEAMED SWEET POTATOES WITH JAPANESE MISO DRESSING

∞

hese potatoes are mild and creamy and just a little tangy. They are delicious with a bowl of steamed jasmine or rose rice and Asian Sweet Pickled Cucumbers (see page 123).

MAKES 4 SERVINGS

> 2 lbs. sweet potatoes, peeled and cut into 2″ chunks
> 2 tablespoons white miso paste*
> 1 teaspoon brown sugar
> 2 tablespoons mirin*
> 1 teaspoon honey
> 1 teaspoon white or white wine vinegar
> ¼ teaspoon toasted sesame oil*

Steam sweet potatoes until fork-tender, about 15–20 minutes. Whisk together remaining ingredients in a large bowl until smooth. Add potatoes to dressing and toss well to coat. Refrigerate until cool.

*See **Specialty Ingredients** (page 34)

NUTRIENT ANALYSIS PER SERVING:
Calories (kcal) 267.54

Protein (g) 4.76	Calories from Protein 18.69	% Calories from Protein 6.98
Carbohydrates (g) 60.08	Calories from Carbohydrates 235.74	% Calories from Carbohydrates 88.11
Fat (g) 1.49	Calories from Fat 13.11	% Calories from Fat 4.90
Saturated Fat (g) 0.26	Total Dietary Fiber (g) 7.27	Sodium (mg) 343.34

JAPANESE-STYLE
STEAMED FRESH SOYBEANS

∞

*F*resh soybeans, or edamame, are a fun and tasty snack to eat right out of hand. They're a *delicious, high protein accompaniment to any Asian meal.*

MAKES 4 SERVINGS

2 cups fresh or frozen soybeans, shelled or in the pod
1 teaspoon toasted sesame seeds lightly ground with ½ teaspoon salt*

Steam soybeans just until tender, about 5 minutes if shelled and 8 minutes if in the pod. Sprinkle lightly with sesame salt and serve.

*See **Specialty Ingredients** (page 34)

NUTRIENT ANALYSIS PER SERVING:
Calories (kcal) 130.68

Protein (g) 11.23	Calories from Protein 41.89	% Calories from Protein 32.06
Carbohydrates(g) 10.12	Calories from Carbohydrates 37.75	% Calories from Carbohydrates 28.89
Fat (g) 6.08	Calories from Fat 51.04	% Calories from Fat 39.06
Saturated Fat (g) 0.71	Total Dietary Fiber (g) 3.89	Sodium (mg) 303.54

ASIAN SWEET PICKLED CUCUMBERS
∞

*T*hese cucumbers make a crunchy, sweet-and-sour side dish that is fabulous with any Asian meal. Although the dressing can be made well in advance, don't add the cucumber itself until just before serving or it will lose its snap.

MAKES 3-4 SERVINGS

> 1 cup white or rice vinegar
> 1 cup granulated sugar
> 1 teaspoon salt
> 1 large cucumber (about 1 lb.)
>
> Cooked jasmine rice for serving

Combine vinegar, sugar, and salt in small saucepan over high heat. Bring to a boil, and cook for 1–2 minutes until slightly reduced and thickened. Chill. Peel cucumber and slice in half lengthwise, scraping out any seeds. Cut halved cucumber crosswise into thin slices, and add to chilled vinegar dressing. Serve immediately with jasmine rice and Barbecued Vietnamese Calamari (page 176), Broiled Red Snapper with Piquant Tamarind Glaze (page 178), Wok-Steamed Teriyaki Ginger Salmon (page 182), Lacquered Five-Spice Chicken (page 195), Thai Grilled Chicken Satays (page 198), or Japanese Soba Noodles with Bonito Dipping Sauce (page 214).

NUTRIENT ANALYSIS PER SERVING:
Calories (kcal) 210.30

Protein (g) 0.40	Calories from Protein 1.50	% Calories from Protein 0.71
Carbohydrates(g) 55.24	Calories from Carbohydrates 207.85	% Calories from Carbohydrates 98.84
Fat (g) 0.11	Calories from Fat 0.95	% Calories from Fat 0.45
Saturated Fat (g) 0.03	Total Dietary Fiber (g) 0.49	Sodium (mg) 583.87

MAPLE-GLAZED RED CABBAGE
∞

*T*his is one of my favorite winter side dishes. Cooking the cabbage makes the insoluble fiber much more tolerable, and served with a high-soluble-fiber main dish it is a delicious accompaniment. I love it with sandwiches and traditional roasted turkey dinners.

MAKES **4-5** SERVINGS

> 2 teaspoons canola oil
> 3 shallots, chopped
> ½ cup maple syrup
> 1 tablespoon brown sugar
> 3 tablespoons balsamic vinegar
> 4 whole cloves
> ½ large head red cabbage, outer leaves discarded, cored, finely shredded
> ¼ teaspoon salt

Heat oil over medium heat in large heavy saucepan. Add shallots and cook until translucent. Add all remaining ingredients. Increase heat to medium high and cook, uncovered, stirring occasionally, until cabbage wilts, about 15 minutes. Cover and cook over medium low until cabbage is tender and limp, about 30 minutes, stirring frequently.

Serve with Simple Herb Baked Chicken Breasts (page 196) and Old-Fashioned Bread Stuffing with Dried Apricots and Currants (page 130).

NUTRIENT ANALYSIS PER SERVING:
Calories (kcal) 177.50

Protein (g) 2.16	Calories from Protein 8.03	% Calories from Protein 4.53
Carbohydrates(g) 39.25	Calories from Carbohydrates 146.11	% Calories from Carbohydrates 82.32
Fat (g) 2.79	Calories from Fat 23.35	% Calories from Fat 13.16
Saturated Fat (g) 0.23	Total Dietary Fiber (g) 2.83	Sodium (mg) 166.37

BASIC ROSE RICE

*R*ose rice is delicious with *Asian* foods, and it makes the creamiest rice puddings imaginable.

MAKES 4 SERVINGS

2 cups rose rice

3 cups water

Put rice in a large saucepan and rinse in several changes of water. Drain. Add the 3 cups water and bring to a boil, uncovered, over high heat. Reduce heat to low, cover, and simmer until rice is tender and cooked through, about 20 minutes. Alternatively, rice can be made in a rice cooker according to manufacturer's instructions.

NUTRIENT ANALYSIS PER SERVING:

Calories (kcal) 342.25

Protein (g) 6.30	Calories from Protein 25.97	% Calories from Protein 7.59
Carbohydrates(g) 75.55	Calories from Carbohydrates 311.56	% Calories from Carbohydrates 91.03
Fat (g) 0.51	Calories from Fat 4.72	% Calories from Fat 1.38
Saturated Fat (g) 0.10	Total Dietary Fiber (g) 2.59	Sodium (mg) 6.47

BASIC JASMINE RICE
∞

*J*asmine rice is wonderful with *Asian foods, seafood, and barbecued chicken.*

MAKES **4** SERVINGS

> 2 cups jasmine rice
> 3 cups water

Put rice in a large saucepan and rinse in several changes of water. Drain. Add the 3 cups water and bring to a boil, uncovered, over high heat. Reduce heat to low, cover, and simmer until rice is tender and cooked through, about 20 minutes. Alternatively, rice can be made in a rice cooker according to manufacturer's instructions.

NUTRIENT ANALYSIS PER SERVING:
Calories (kcal) 337.63

Protein (g) 6.60	Calories from Protein 27.18	% Calories from Protein 8.05
Carbohydrates(g) 73.95	Calories from Carbohydrates 304.78	% Calories from Carbohydrates 90.27
Fat (g) 0.61	Calories from Fat 5.66	% Calories from Fat 1.68
Saturated Fat (g) 0.17	Total Dietary Fiber (g) 1.20	Sodium (mg) 4.63

BASIC BASMATI RICE
∞

*B*asmati rice is the best choice for *Middle Eastern and Indian dishes. It has a chewy texture and slightly nutty flavor that has no substitute.*

MAKES **4** SERVINGS

> 2 cups basmati rice
> 3 cups water

Put rice in a large saucepan and rinse in several changes of water. Drain. Add the 3 cups water and bring to a boil, uncovered, over high heat. Reduce heat to low, cover, and simmer until rice is tender and cooked through, about 20 minutes. Alternatively, rice can be made in a rice cooker according to manufacturer's instructions.

NUTRIENT ANALYSIS PER SERVING:
Calories (kcal) 351.00

Protein (g) 6.44	Calories from Protein 26.59	% Calories from Protein 7.58
Carbohydrates(g) 77.36	Calories from Carbohydrates 319.16	% Calories from Carbohydrates 90.93
Fat (g) 0.57	Calories from Fat 5.25	% Calories from Fat 1.50
Saturated Fat (g) 0.15	Total Dietary Fiber (g) 1.36	Sodium (mg) 0.98

BASIC BROWN RICE
∽

*B*rown rice is wonderful with grilled salmon and all types of vegetarian meals. Try a bowl plain with a splash of fresh lemon juice and a sprinkle of garlic salt for a quick, tasty, and safe snack.

MAKES 6 SERVINGS

> 2 cups brown rice
> 4 cups water

Put rice in a large saucepan and rinse in several changes of water. Drain. Add the 4 cups water and bring to a boil, uncovered, over high heat. Reduce heat to low, cover, and simmer until rice is tender and cooked through, about 40 minutes. Alternatively, rice can be made in a rice cooker according to manufacturer's instructions.

NUTRIENT ANALYSIS PER SERVING:
Calories (kcal) 229.27

Protein (g) 4.75	Calories from Protein 19.17	% Calories from Protein 8.36
Carbohydrates(g) 48.24	Calories from Carbohydrates 194.68	% Calories from Carbohydrates 84.92
Fat (g) 1.70	Calories from Fat 15.41	% Calories from Fat 6.72
Saturated Fat (g) 0.34	Total Dietary Fiber (g) 2.15	odium (mg) 2.53

SWEET CARDAMOM
AND CURRANT INDIAN RICE
∞

*I*love this rice with Indian Curried Potatoes, Peas and Carrots (page 210). It provides a sweet and subtle fruit-and-nut counterbalance to that headily-seasoned dish. The scent of the cardamom in this recipe will perfume your entire house as it cooks.

MAKES 6 SERVINGS

2 cups white basmati rice*
3 cups water
2 cinnamon sticks
10 whole cloves
1/4 teaspoon salt

1/2 cup water
1 cup brown sugar
2 teaspoons ground cardamom (freshly ground from seeds, if possible)

2 teaspoons canola oil
1/2 cup slivered almonds
1/2 cup diced raisins

Place rice in electric rice cooker or large saucepan and rinse thoroughly with cold water until water runs clear. Drain. Add 3 cups water, cinnamon sticks, cloves, and salt. Cook in rice cooker or bring to boil over stove, reduce heat to low, cover, and simmer for 20 minutes undisturbed. Set aside.

In a small saucepan over medium high heat combine 1/2 cup water, sugar, and cardamom. Heat until mixture boils and reduces slightly to a syrup. Pour over cooked rice. Stir thoroughly and let sit uncovered if rice is wet.

In small non-stick skillet heat oil. Add almonds and raisins and fry over medium heat, stirring constantly, until almonds turn golden and raisins puff. Gently stir into rice and serve.

*Basmati rice is available at grocery stores, Indian markets, Middle Eastern markets, or see Directory of Resources.

NUTRIENT ANALYSIS PER SERVING:
Calories (kcal) 433.46

Protein (g) 6.66	Calories from Protein 26.33	% Calories from Protein 6.07
Carbohydrates(g) 85.16	Calories from Carbohydrates 336.44	% Calories from Carbohydrates 77.62
Fat (g) 7.95	Calories from Fat 70.69	% Calories from Fat 16.31
Saturated Fat (g) 0.80	Total Dietary Fiber (g) 2.86	Sodium (mg) 112.12

RAISIN BREAD ROSEMARY STUFFING

∾

I love stuffings, and this is one of my favorites. It has a delicious combination of flavors, and with some tender steamed green vegetables and Simple Herb Baked Chicken Breasts (page 196), it makes a great fast dinner.

MAKES 8-10 SERVINGS

2 cups onion, finely chopped
2 tablespoons canola oil
1 cup finely chopped fresh cranberries
2 tablespoons packed brown sugar
2 teaspoons dried rosemary, crushed
½ teaspoon dried sage
7 cups raisin bread, cut into ½" cubes and toasted (about 12 slices)
½ cup fresh orange juice
½ cup vegetable or fat-free chicken broth
Salt and pepper, to taste

Preheat oven to 325°F. In a large non-stick skillet cook the onion in the oil over medium heat until softened. Add cranberries, brown sugar, rosemary, sage, and salt and pepper to taste. Cook, stirring, for 5 minutes. Transfer mixture to a large bowl, add toasted bread cubes and orange juice, and stir gently but thoroughly until well-combined. Spoon stuffing into a 3–quart casserole dish, drizzle with the broth, and bake, covered, for 30 minutes. Uncover and bake 30 minutes more.

NUTRIENT ANALYSIS PER SERVING:
Calories (kcal) 197.57

Protein (g) 4.37	Calories from Protein 16.92	% Calories from Protein 8.57
Carbohydrates(g) 33.76	Calories from Carbohydrates 130.85	% Calories from Carbohydrates 66.23
Fat (g) 5.71	Calories from Fat 49.79	% Calories from Fat 25.20
Saturated Fat (g) 0.78	Total Dietary Fiber (g) 3.37	Sodium (mg) 186.82

OLD-FASHIONED BREAD STUFFING WITH DRIED APRICOTS AND CURRANTS

∞

This is a terrific stuffing for a Thanksgiving turkey, a roasted chicken, or Cornish game hens. I also serve it with Candied Sweet Potatoes (page 119) and steamed fresh green beans for a very satisfying vegetarian meal.

MAKES 6 SERVINGS

2 tablespoons olive oil
2 large shallots, minced
1 medium onion, minced
2 garlic cloves, minced
½ teaspoon sage
⅛ teaspoon cloves
⅛ teaspoon crushed rosemary
¼ teaspoon marjoram
¼ teaspoon savory
¼ garlic salt
⅓ cup currants, chopped
¼ cup celery, finely chopped
½ cup dried apricots, finely chopped
½ cup white wine
4 whole sourdough English muffins, toasted, cooled, torn into small bite size pieces*
Vegetable broth, if needed
Salt and pepper, to taste

Preheat oven to 325°F. In large heavy non-stick skillet heat the oil over medium heat, add shallots, onion, and garlic. Cook, stirring, until vegetables are golden. Stir in spices, currants, celery, and apricots. Cook, stirring, for 1 minute. Add wine and simmer until most but not all of the liquid evaporates. Remove from heat and stir in bread pieces and salt and pepper to taste. If stuffing looks too dry drizzle with a few tablespoons of vegetable broth.

Place stuffing in a non-stick 9 x 5" loaf pan, cover with foil, and bake for one hour.

*English muffins give the perfect texture to this stuffing.

NUTRIENT ANALYSIS PER SERVING:

Calories (kcal) 175.74

Protein (g) 3.70	Calories from Protein 15.71	% Calories from Protein 8.94
Carbohydrates(g) 25.81	Calories from Carbohydrates 109.54	% Calories from Carbohydrates 62.33
Fat (g) 5.29	Calories from Fat 50.49	% Calories from Fat 28.73
Saturated Fat (g) 0.72	Total Dietary Fiber (g)* 2.13	Sodium (mg) 280.42

TUSCAN TOMATO BREAD SALAD

∞

*H*ere's the perfect salad for fresh ripe tomatoes and basil from your summer garden. Bread salad is a country Italian staple, and it makes a rustic, delicious, and safe meal.

MAKES 3-4 SERVINGS

DRESSING:

1 tablespoon extra virgin olive oil

3 tablespoons white or red wine vinegar

1 tablespoon balsamic vinegar

1 small garlic clove, minced to a paste with a dash of salt

Salt and white pepper to taste

SALAD:

3 cups stale crusty French or Italian bread, cut into ½" cubes
½ lb. fresh ripe tomatoes, diced
1 small cucumber, peeled, seeded, and diced
1 cup thinly sliced red onions
½ cup packed basil leaves, stems removed, finely shredded

Whisk together all dressing ingredients and set aside.

Combine all salad ingredients in a large bowl and toss gently. Drizzle with dressing and toss to coat.

NUTRIENT ANALYSIS PER SERVING:
Calories (kcal) 304.63

Protein (g) 8.65	Calories from Protein 34.11	% Calories from Protein 11.20
Carbohydrates(g) 51.95	Calories from Carbohydrates 204.92	% Calories from Carbohydrates 67.27
Fat (g) 7.39	Calories from Fat 65.60	% Calories from Fat 21.53
Saturated Fat (g) 1.20	Total Dietary Fiber (g) 4.39	Sodium (mg) 508.93

TANGY THAI SALAD WITH FRESH HERBS

When it's too hot to cook, this salad makes a light and delicious one-dish meal. Please don't be afraid of the TVP—it's easy to find at health food stores, it's a nutritional power-house, and it will absorb the flavors you add to it. It's also very high in soluble fiber and makes a great base for the vegetables in the recipe. I have had people think this salad was made from ground pork, ground chicken, or ground shrimp—the TVP makes a completely convincing substitute for all three. For a refreshing accompaniment, try chilled glasses of Spring Blossom Tea (page 44).

MAKES 8 SERVINGS

Add the following to a large bowl and let stand for 10–15 minutes, stirring occasionally:

2 cups TVP (textured vegetable protein, a soy product)*
2 cups boiling water
Juice of 2 limes
¼ cup Thai or Vietnamese fish sauce*

Add to TVP mixture and stir thoroughly:

2 scallions, diced
2 stalks of fresh lemongrass, lower three inches trimmed and finely minced*
1 small bunch fresh basil leaves, stems removed, finely shredded
1 small bunch fresh mint leaves, stems removed, finely shredded
1 large sweet potato, peeled, diced, and steamed or microwaved until fork-tender
½ medium onion, diced
3 tablespoons Thai fried red onions or shallots*

Make dressing by stirring together the following 4 ingredients until sugar dissolves:

Juice of 2 limes
¼ teaspoon cayenne, or to taste
1 tablespoon brown sugar
2 tablespoons Thai or Vietnamese fish sauce*

Fresh Napa cabbage leaves, washed, bottom ends trimmed and discarded, for serving

Add dressing to TVP mixture, stirring well. Let sit for 30–60 minutes to develop flavors. Have people serve themselves by spooning a generous amount of salad mixture onto individual cabbage leaves and rolling up to eat.

*See **Specialty Ingredients** (page 34)

NUTRIENT ANALYSIS PER SERVING:
Calories (kcal) 141.85

Protein (g) 16.26	Calories from Protein 60.47	% Calories from Protein 42.63
Carbohydrates(g) 20.12	Calories from Carbohydrates 74.81	% Calories from Carbohydrates 52.74
Fat (g) 0.79	Calories from Fat 6.57	% Calories from Fat 4.63
Saturated Fat (g) 0.09	Total Dietary Fiber (g) 0.90	Sodium (mg) 1046.89

RICE NOODLE SALAD
WITH SHRIMP AND MANGO
∞

ave one taste and you'll see why this is one of my very favorite salads. The dressing is tart and tangy, the shrimp and mango mellow and sweet, and the colors absolutely gorgeous. Rice noodles are a great staple for so many recipes, but this is truly one of the best.

MAKES 3 SERVINGS

DRESSING:

2 tablespoons Thai or Vietnamese fish sauce*
1 tablespoon white vinegar
1 tablespoon granulated sugar
2 tablespoons fresh lime juice
1 large garlic clove, minced

Combine all dressing ingredients in a small bowl and set aside.

SALAD:

½ lb. shrimp, shelled and deveined
½ lb. flat, ¼" dry rice noodles**
½ cup peeled, diced, seeded cucumber
½ cup thinly sliced sweet white onion, such as Maui or Walla Walla
3 tablespoons packed fresh cilantro leaves, stems removed, finely chopped
3 tablespoons packed fresh mint leaves, stems removed, finely chopped
½ small ripe mango, peeled and diced

In a large saucepan of boiling water cook shrimp until just pink and cooked through, about 2 minutes. Drain. Halve shrimp horizontally and roughly chop.

In a bowl soak rice noodles in hot water to cover 15 minutes to soften. While noodles soak, bring a large saucepan of water to boil. Add drained noodles and cook in boiling water just until tender, about 1 minute. Drain noodles and rinse with cold water until cool.

Combine noodles, shrimp, dressing, and all remaining ingredients in a large bowl. Toss until thoroughly mixed, then divide among 3 serving bowls.

*See **Specialty Ingredients** (page 34)
**Available at Asian markets, or see Directory of Resources

NUTRIENT ANALYSIS PER SERVING:
Calories (kcal) 219.27

Protein (g) 17.45	Calories from Protein 69.97	% Calories from Protein 31.91
Carbohydrates(g) 33.50	Calories from Carbohydrates 134.36	% Calories from Carbohydrates 61.27
Fat (g) 1.66	Calories from Fat 14.94	% Calories from Fat 6.81
Saturated Fat (g) 0.31	Cholesterol (mg) 114.84	Total Dietary Fiber (g) 2.15
Sodium (mg) 1059.46		

ROASTED SWEET POTATO CIDER SALAD

∞

This is a delicious twist on traditional potato salad, and it is incredibly simple to make. The sweetness of the potatoes plays off the tanginess of the cider vinegar, with truly delectable results.

MAKES 4 SERVINGS

1½ pounds sweet potatoes (about 2 large), peeled, quartered lengthwise
1 tablespoon plus 1 teaspoon olive oil, divided
2 tablespoons scallions, finely diced
3 tablespoons apple cider vinegar
⅛ teaspoon salt

Preheat oven to 400°F. Place sweet potatoes in large baking dish, drizzle with 1 tablespoon oil, and toss potatoes until evenly coated. Cover pan with foil and bake 20 minutes. Uncover pan, turn potatoes and bake uncovered until tender and golden brown, about 15–20 minutes. Cool potatoes and chop into bite-size pieces. Transfer to serving bowl.

Whisk vinegar with remaining teaspoon of oil and salt. Pour over potatoes, add scallions, and stir gently until well combined.

NUTRIENT ANALYSIS PER SERVING:
Calories (kcal) 220.92

Protein (g) 2.86	Calories from Protein 11.22	% Calories from Protein 5.08
Carbohydrates(g) 42.18	Calories from Carbohydrates 165.44	% Calories from Carbohydrates 74.89
Fat (g) 5.02	Calories from Fat 44.26	% Calories from Fat 20.03
Saturated Fat (g) 0.72	Total Dietary Fiber (g) 5.18	Sodium (mg) 95.38
Sodium (mg) 223.42		

SUMMER CHICKEN, NEW POTATO, AND GREEN BEAN SALAD

∞

*T*his salad makes a light and delicious variation of a traditional summer standby. The soluble fiber of the potatoes and low fat level of the dressing make it just as safe as it is appetizing. Serve it at your next backyard picnic, then stand back and wait for the applause.

MAKES 4 SERVINGS

> 3 cups water (or 1½ cups water plus 1½ cups white wine)
> 2 organic skinless, boneless chicken breasts
> 1 medium onion, thinly sliced
> 10 whole peppercorns
> 1 teaspoon garlic salt

Add all ingredients to a medium saucepan and bring to boil. Poach chicken, covered, over medium low heat for 10–15 minutes until cooked through. Remove from heat and cool chicken in broth to room temperature. Drain and discard cooking liquid and onion, and tear chicken into small pieces. Set aside.

> 1½ lbs. small red or white new potatoes, scrubbed
> 1 teaspoon garlic salt
> ½ lb. fresh green beans, trimmed, cut into 1" lengths
> ½ cup sun-dried tomatoes (not in oil)
> 1 small red onion, thinly sliced
> 2 tablespoons fresh lemon juice
> ¼ cup balsamic vinegar
> 2 tablespoons Dijon mustard
> 1 teaspoon rosemary, crushed
> 1 teaspoon oregano
> ¼ cup fresh basil leaves, washed, stems removed, finely shredded
> 1 tablespoon olive oil
>
> Fresh crusty French bread for serving

Cut potatoes in half and add to a large saucepan. Cover with cold water by one inch, add garlic salt, and bring to boil. Cook for 10–12 minutes, or until fork-tender. Use a slotted spoon to remove potatoes to a colander and rinse with cold water. Add the green beans to cooking water, cook 3–5 minutes until tender. Drain in colander with potatoes. Dice sun-dried tomatoes (soften in hot water first if necessary). Whisk together remaining ingredients to form dressing. In a large bowl combine chicken, potatoes, green beans, tomatoes, and dressing. Add salt and pepper to taste. Serve with crusty French bread.

NUTRIENT ANALYSIS PER SERVING:
Calories (kcal) 343.98

Protein (g) 33.20	Calories from Protein 130.64	% Calories from Protein 37.98
Carbohydrates(g) 42.20	Calories from Carbohydrates 166.08	% Calories from Carbohydrates 48.28
Fat (g) 5.34	Calories from Fat 47.26	% Calories from Fat 13.74
Saturated Fat (g) 0.94	Cholesterol (mg) 68.44	Total Dietary Fiber (g) 6.14
Sodium (mg) 814.18		

ITALIAN TUNA, LEMON, AND BASIL PASTA SALAD

∞

a wonderful one-dish meal on a hot summer day. This salad combines bright, festive colors and traditional Italian flavors, plus a high soluble fiber foundation of pasta.

MAKES 3 SERVINGS (EASILY DOUBLED)

SALAD:

8 oz. spaghetti, cooked until tender, drained, and rinsed with cold water
2 tablespoons finely shredded fresh basil leaves
2 tablespoons finely chopped scallions
1 medium fresh ripe tomato, diced
¼ cup diced white onion
6 oz. can of solid white albacore tuna
Salt and pepper to taste

DRESSING:

Juice from 2 lemons
1 tablespoon extra virgin olive oil
1¼ teaspoon dried parsley
1¼ teaspoon dillweed
1 small clove garlic, minced and mashed to a paste with a dash of salt

Whisk together all dressing ingredients. Combine salad ingredients in two serving bowls and lightly toss to combine. Drizzle dressing over salad and serve.

NUTRIENT ANALYSIS PER SERVING:
Calories (kcal) 415.85

Protein (g) 23.74	Calories from Protein 95.63	% Calories from Protein 23.00
Carbohydrates(g) 62.53	Calories from Carbohydrates 251.88	% Calories from Carbohydrates 60.57
Fat (g) 7.54	Calories from Fat 68.34	% Calories from Fat 16.43
Saturated Fat (g) 1.25	Cholesterol (mg) 23.80	Total Dietary Fiber (g) 2.59

SOUPS AND
SANDWICHES

∞

Soups and sandwiches are among the quickest, tastiest foods to make following the IBS diet, and they both offer great ways to add lots of fresh vegetables to a soluble fiber base. For most soups, the only modifications needed are the substitution of soy milk for cream-based broths in chowders or bisques, and the addition of high soluble fiber foods like rice, potatoes, carrots, turnips, or other root vegetables. Make sure to simmer your soups until all the vegetables are quite tender, and remember that you can purée them as well to further minimize the insoluble fiber. Replace high fat chicken or beef stock with low fat vegetable broth, and top your soups with homemade croutons or fat-free crackers for additional soluble fiber.

For sandwiches, using French or sourdough bread provides a built-in soluble fiber base and gives you the perfect opportunity to incorporate a variety of fresh produce. Stick to low fat poultry or seafood choices, use flavorful chutneys, bean spreads, or marinades instead of high fat dressings, and add in a medley of finely sliced vegetables.

You just can't beat soups and sandwiches for fast, delicious lunches, and all of the choices in this chapter pack well for a brown bag treat at work or your next road trip picnic. Add in some baked potato chips or pretzels, a slice or two of homemade fruit bread, and a small fresh peeled pear or apple for dessert, and you've got yourself a safe, tasty lunch in a flash.

BASIC VEGETABLE STOCK

∞

*I*t's fast and easy to make your own stock, and the results are so much better than the canned versions. You can freeze stock in small containers to use as needed.

MAKES 2¹/₂ QUARTS

I lb. leeks, washed very well, diced
1½ lbs. carrots, diced
1½ lbs. onions, diced
2 tablespoons olive oil
2 bay leaves
2 teaspoons thyme
I large bunch fresh flat-leaf parsley
3 quarts water

In a large stock pot heat oil over medium low heat. Add vegetables and sauté, stirring occasionally, until softened but not brown, about 5–10 minutes. Add herbs and water and bring to a boil. Reduce heat and simmer, covered, skimming as necessary, about 45 minutes. Strain and cool.

Stock freezes up to 3 months.

NUTRIENT ANALYSIS PER RECIPE:
Calories (kcal) 238.68
Fat (g) 27.00   Calories from Fat 238.68   % Calories from Fat 100.00
Saturated Fat (g) 3.65   Sodium (mg) 0.01

SMOKY SWEET POTATO SOUP

∞

*T*his soup is one of my all-time favorite Mexican recipes. It is sweet, smoky, earthy goodness in a bowl. It's impressive enough for guests, yet easy enough for a throw-together workweek dinner.

MAKES **8** SERVINGS

> 1½ lbs. sweet potatoes, peeled and diced (about 3 medium)
> 4 carrots, peeled and diced
> 6 cups vegetable broth
> 1 teaspoon dried thyme
> 2 teaspoons canola oil
> 1 cup finely diced onion
> 4 garlic cloves, minced
> 2 teaspoons maple syrup
> 2 teaspoons honey
> 1–3 teaspoons chipotle powder, to taste*
>
> Fresh cilantro leaves, stems removed, finely shredded, for serving
> Baked corn chips (Tostitos), for serving

In a large heavy stockpot simmer the sweet potatoes, carrots, thyme, and broth for 2 hours, covered, stirring occasionally with a wire whisk, until vegetables disintegrate. Mash vegetables in pot with a potato masher if necessary.

In a non-stick skillet heat oil over medium low, and sauté onion and garlic until lightly golden. Add to broth with maple syrup, honey, and chipotle powder to taste. Serve individual bowls of soup topped with a sprinkle of cilantro. Serve with baked corn chips.

*See **Specialty Ingredients** (page 34)

NUTRIENT ANALYSIS PER SERVING:
Calories (kcal) 130.86

Protein (g) 2.10	Calories from Protein 8.12	% Calories from Protein 6.21
Carbohydrates(g) 28.24	Calories from Carbohydrates 109.45	% Calories from Carbohydrates 83.64
Fat (g) 1.52	Calories from Fat 13.28	% Calories from Fat 10.15
Saturated Fat (g) 0.15	Total Dietary Fiber (g) 3.98	Sodium (mg) 26.05

COUNTRY TOMATO ONION SOUP WITH BASIL PARMESAN CROUTONS

∽

*S*imple to make, and simply delicious to eat. This is one my favorite childhood soups. It's mild, comforting, and comes together in a flash from ingredients you're likely to have on hand. Just don't skimp on the croutons, as they provide the soluble fiber that makes this a safe meal—and they're also the tastiest part!

MAKES 8 SERVINGS

SOUP:

2 tablespoons olive oil
4 large yellow onions, thinly sliced
5 large garlic cloves, minced
1 tablespoon all-purpose unbleached white flour
1½ teaspoons salt
4 cups vegetable stock or water
1 (1 lb, 12 oz) can tomatoes, whole or chopped, undrained, puréed in blender until smooth

BASIL PARMESAN CROUTONS:

16 large slices French bread, lightly toasted
1 cup packed fresh basil leaves
4 tablespoons olive oil
2 tablespoons soy Parmesan

Heat the oil over medium heat in a large stock pot, and add the onions. Sauté, stirring occasionally until golden, about 45 minutes. Add the garlic and sift in the flour and cook another 15 minutes. Stir in the salt and water, bring to a boil, then reduce heat and simmer, covered, for 15 minutes. Add the tomato purée and simmer 10–15 minutes more.

Preheat oven to 350°F. In a blender purée the basil and oil until liquified. In a large baking pan toss bread with basil oil and bake, shaking pan occasionally, for 10–15 minutes or until croutons are golden brown and crisp (flip once for even baking). Remove from oven and sprinkle with soy Parmesan.

To serve, place a crouton into each bowl, ladle in soup, and top each bowl with another crouton.

NUTRIENT ANALYSIS PER SERVING:
Calories (kcal) 281.46

Protein (g) 8.24	Calories from Protein 32.57	% Calories from Protein 11.57
Carbohydrates(g) 48.77	Calories from Carbohydrates 192.67	% Calories from Carbohydrates 68.45
Fat (g) 6.32	Calories from Fat 56.23	% Calories from Fat 19.98
Saturated Fat (g) 1.02	Total Dietary Fiber (g) 4.55	Sodium (mg) 871.83

NEW ENGLAND CLAM CHOWDER
∞

I have loved clam chowder since childhood, but the traditional cream-based recipe just kills me. Here, with the easy substitution of soy or rice milk for dairy, my favorite soup becomes perfectly safe, not to mention simply delicious.

MAKES 6 SERVINGS

I tablespoon olive oil
I large onion, diced
2 large carrots, scraped and diced
½ cup all-purpose unbleached white flour
2 cups clam broth
3 cups plain soy or rice milk
2 6.5 oz. cans chopped or minced clams
½ teaspoon white pepper
I tablespoon dried parsley
¾ teaspoon salt
½ teaspoon crushed thyme
I bay leaf
¼ teaspoon ground black pepper
4 cups Russet baking potatoes (about 2 large), peeled and diced into I″ cubes

Salt and pepper to taste for serving

Fat-free saltines for serving

In a large stockpot heat the oil over medium heat. Add the onions and carrots and sauté until softened. Gradually sift in the flour, stirring thoroughly and scraping bottom of pan. Very gradually stir in the clam broth, scraping sides and bottom of pan to make sure flour is thoroughly incorporated without clumping. Stir in soy or rice milk until mixture is smooth. Add the clams and spices, bring soup to a boil, then cover and reduce heat. Simmer for 30 minutes. Add diced potatoes, cover and simmer for an additional 30 minutes. Taste and adjust seasoning with salt and pepper. Serve with crushed saltines.

NUTRIENT ANALYSIS PER SERVING:

Calories (kcal) 249.19

Protein (g) 21.72	Calories from Protein 86.87	% Calories from Protein 34.86
Carbohydrates(g) 27.08	Calories from Carbohydrates 108.30	% Calories from Carbohydrates 43.46
Fat (g) 6.00	Calories from Fat 54.02	% Calories from Fat 21.68
Saturated Fat (g) 0.72	Cholesterol (mg) 41.13	Total Dietary Fiber (g) 3.68
Sodium (mg) 290.20		

MOROCCAN CHICKPEA AND BREAD PEASANT STEW WITH HARISSA

∞

*I*f you've never had Moroccan food before, you are in for a real treat with this stew. It's half bread, half tender seasoned chickpeas, and wholly delicious. The harissa, a traditional North African condiment, is worth the extra effort as it lends an authentic and special smoky flavor to the meal. Ready-made harissa can also be found at some specialty and ethnic stores, though it may be hotter than the recipe included here.

MAKES 8 SERVINGS

12 cups water
1 pound dried chickpeas (about 2⅓ cups)
1 very large onion, diced
12 large garlic cloves, minced
2 teaspoons harissa (optional, but really delicious)
2 teaspoons whole cumin seeds
2 teaspoons whole caraway seeds
1 tablespoon salt
1 loaf French bread, torn into bite-size chunks
Fresh lemon slices for serving
Chopped capers for serving

HARISSA:

5 oz. dried New Mexico chiles (about 20)*
¾ teaspoon freshly ground dry-roasted caraway seeds
2 teaspoons freshly ground dry-roasted coriander seeds
1 small garlic clove, minced
¾ teaspoon salt
3 tablespoons extra virgin olive oil

Stem and seed dried chiles and cover with boiling water until softened, about 1 hour. Drain. In a food processor blend chiles and all remaining ingredients. Discard any pieces of chile skins that will not blend in. Pack harissa into a small jar and freeze to store (will keep for months).

In a large stock pot combine water, chickpeas, onion, and garlic. Bring to a boil, cover, and simmer mixture until chickpeas are tender, about 2 hours. While chickpeas are cooking, heat a large skillet (not non-stick) without oil over medium high heat. Add the cumin and caraway seeds and toast until they are fragrant but not smoking. Cool seeds and grind to a fine powder in blender, spice grinder, or coffee grinder.

Add ground spices, harissa, and salt to chickpeas. Cook another 30 minutes, occasionally mashing down the chickpeas with a potato masher. You may purée the soup in a blender if you wish, or simply keep cooking it until the chickpeas disintegrate.

Cover the bottom of the serving bowls with bread chunks, and ladle the soup on top. Sprinkle a small spoonful of capers over each serving, and squeeze a lemon slice or two on top.

*New Mexico chiles are large, dried red chiles with mild to moderate heat. They are available at many Hispanic or Indian markets, health food stores, or see Directory of Resources.

Nutrient Analysis Per Serving:
Calories (kcal) 385.52

Protein (g) 16.44	Calories from Protein 64.96	% Calories from Protein 6.85
Carbohydrates(g) 66.93	Calories from Carbohydrates 264.50	% Calories from Carbohydrates 68.61
Fat (g) 6.30	Calories from Fat 56.06	% Calories from Fat 14.54
Saturated Fat (g) 0.88	Total Dietary Fiber (g) 12.00	Sodium (mg) 1232.29

ROASTED CAULIFLOWER CARAWAY SOUP

∞

his soup is creamy, hearty, and subtly seasoned. It's a wonderful winter meal in itself, or add a grilled vegetable sandwich for the perfect lunch on a snowy day.

MAKES 4 SERVINGS

1 large head cauliflower, leaves and green stalks removed
6 whole garlic cloves
½ small onion, coarsely chopped
1 tablespoon olive oil
2 cups veggie broth
¼ teaspoon dried thyme
1 bay leaf
1½–2 cups unsweetened soy or rice milk
½ teaspoon salt
1 teaspoon caraway seeds, ground
1 teaspoon cumin seeds, ground
3–4 tablespoons cream sherry, to taste

Fresh rosemary sourdough bread, toasted, for serving

Preheat oven to 425°F. Cut cauliflower into 1″ pieces and place in a large roasting pan with garlic and onion. Drizzle with oil; stir well. Roast in oven for 30 minutes, stirring once halfway through cooking.

In a large heavy stockpot simmer broth over medium low heat with roasted cauliflower mixture, thyme, bay leaf, caraway, cumin, and salt, for 30 minutes, covered, stirring frequently. Remove bay leaf and purée soup in pot with hand-held blender, adding 1 cup of the soy or rice milk to ease blending. Alternately, carefully pour soup into blender or food mill with 1 cup of the soy or rice milk and purée, then return to pot. Add remaining soy or rice milk until thinned as desired, stir in sherry, and heat through on low. Serve with rosemary sourdough bread.

NUTRIENT ANALYSIS PER SERVING:
Calories (kcal) 139.34

Protein (g) 7.47	Calories from Protein 30.14	% Calories from Protein 21.63
Carbohydrates(g) 13.27	Calories from Carbohydrates 53.58	% Calories from Carbohydrates 38.46
Fat (g) 6.12	Calories from Fat 55.61	% Calories from Fat 39.91
Saturated Fat (g) 0.78	Total Dietary Fiber (g) 5.79	Sodium (mg) 336.96

CANTONESE JOK
(RICE PORRIDGE SOUP)

∞

*T*his is probably the single most soothing, safe, and nutritious bowl of soup for people with IBS. It is a wonderful staple and something you might want to make on a weekly basis. Most Chinese people have a bowl for breakfast every morning—not a bad idea at all. The recipe comes from Sifu Winchell Woo, my husband's Kung Fu teacher in Springfield, Massachusetts. Sifu is a renowned chef, and it is quite an honor that he allowed me to use his recipe—so enjoy it!

MAKES 4 SERVINGS (EASILY DOUBLED OR TRIPLED)

I cup jasmine or other long grain white rice, rinsed and drained
⅛ teaspoon baking soda
¼ teaspoon salt
¼ teaspoon peanut or canola oil
¼ teaspoon toasted sesame oil*

FOR SERVING:

Finely chopped scallions
White pepper
Cooked shrimp
Soy sauce (try Jen Mai)
Toasted sesame oil

Put rice in a small bowl and cover with water. Mix in baking soda, salt, and peanut oil. Let stand at room temperature overnight.

In a large stockpot bring 12 (yes, 12) cups water to a boil and add to rice mixture. Cook at a low boil, uncovered, until the mixture starts to thicken. Reduce heat to a bare simmer, add sesame oil, and cook until mixture is the consistency of porridge. Serve plain or topped with scallions, white pepper, cooked shrimp, soy sauce, and sesame oil to taste.

*See **Specialty Ingredients** (page 34)

NUTRIENT ANALYSIS PER SERVING WITHOUT TOPPINGS:
Calories (kcal) 173.90

Protein (g) 3.30	Calories from Protein 13.57	% Calories from Protein 7.80
Carbohydrates(g) 36.98	Calories from Carbohydrates 152.17	% Calories from Carbohydrates 87.51
Fat (g) 0.88	Calories from Fat 8.15	% Calories from Fat 4.69
Saturated Fat (g) 0.14	Total Dietary Fiber (g) 0.60	Sodium (mg) 186.99

CHINESE SWEET CORN AND CRAB VELVET SOUP

∞

*T*his is a safe version of a delicious soup served in almost every Chinese restaurant. Using canned cream corn instead of fresh kernels reduces the insoluble fiber content and accents the subtle sweetness of the crab. This is delicious served over rice or with an assortment of steamed Chinese dumplings from your local Asian market.

MAKES 8 SERVINGS

2 tablespoons plus 2 teaspoons cornstarch
6 cups vegetable or fat-free chicken broth
1 slice fresh gingerroot, finely minced
2 tablespoon mirin* or sherry
1 tablespoon granulated sugar
2 14.5–oz. cans creamed sweet corn (about 2½ cups)
4 organic egg whites, beaten slightly
1 cup crabmeat or surimi*
¼ teaspoon salt

Rose rice for serving (see page 125)

Put the cornstarch in a small bowl and slowly stir in just enough water to make a thin liquid. Set aside.

Heat the broth and add the ginger, mirin, sugar, and corn. Bring to a boil and drizzle in the egg whites, swirling the soup with a spoon as you do so (the egg should cook into long strands in the broth). Add the crab, salt and pepper and gradually stir in the liquified cornstarch until soup slightly thickens. Serve over rice.

*See **Specialty Ingredients** (page 34)

NUTRIENT ANALYSIS PER SERVING:
Calories (kcal) 80.39

Protein (g) 5.86	Calories from Protein 22.34	% Calories from Protein 27.79
Carbohydrates(g) 14.02	Calories from Carbohydrates 53.49	% Calories from Carbohydrates 66.55
Fat (g) 0.53	Calories from Fat 4.55	% Calories from Fat 5.66
Saturated Fat (g) 0.08	Cholesterol (mg) 14.75	Total Dietary Fiber (g) 0.77
Sodium (mg) 323.85		

SANDWICHES OF SESAME CHICKEN AND ASIAN COLESLAW

*T*his recipe is a great change of pace when you're tired of the same old chicken sandwich.

MAKES 4 SANDWICHES

1½ tablespoons all-purpose unbleached white flour
2 tablespoons toasted sesame seeds*
1 organic egg white
1 teaspoon water
1 pound organic boneless, skinless chicken breasts, halved horizontally and flattened
2 teaspoons toasted sesame oil
1 tablespoon fresh lemon juice
2 cups finely shredded Napa cabbage
1 carrot, finely shredded
1 tablespoon rice wine vinegar

Two 12″ long narrow French bread baguettes, halved horizontally, toasted

Add flour to one dinner plate, and add sesame seeds to a separate dinner plate. Whisk together egg white and water in a small bowl. Coat chicken breasts with flour, shaking off excess, then dip in egg mixture, and coat with sesame seeds.

Heat a large non-stick skillet over medium heat and add 1 teaspoon sesame oil. Add chicken and cook until golden, about 4–5 minutes. Turn chicken and cook another 4–5 minutes, or until just cooked through. Add lemon juice to pan, turn chicken to coat with juice, and cook an additional minute until juice evaporates.

In a medium bowl toss together cabbage, carrot, remaining teaspoon sesame oil, vinegar, and salt and pepper to taste.

Make sandwiches on the toasted baguettes with the chicken and coleslaw.

*See **Specialty Ingredients** (page 34)

NUTRIENT ANALYSIS PER SERVING:
Calories (kcal) 390.98
Protein (g) 34.89
Carbohydrates(g) 43.74
Fat (g) 7.86
Saturated Fat (g) 1.43
Sodium (mg) 524.74

Calories from Protein 141.64
Calories from Carbohydrates 177.54
Calories from Fat 71.81
Cholesterol (mg) 65.77

% Calories from Protein 36.23
% Calories from Carbohydrates 45.41
% Calories from Fat 18.37
Total Dietary Fiber (g) 4.23

SANDWICHES OF TERIYAKI-GRILLED PORTOBELLO MUSHROOMS WITH ASIAN COLESLAW

∞

This is a great vegetarian recipe for people who like meat sandwiches. Portobello mushrooms have a rich, earthy flavor and a very meaty texture that lends itself beautifully to sandwiches. The French bread base allows you to safely add the insoluble fiber of the coleslaw.

MAKES 4 SERVINGS

TERIYAKI MUSHROOMS:

¼ cup soy sauce

2 tablespoons mirin*

3 tablespoons white vinegar

1½ tablespoons minced peeled fresh gingerroot

1 minced garlic clove

2 tablespoons honey

4 fresh Portobello mushrooms (about ¼ lb. each), stems removed

Two 12" long narrow French bread baguettes, halved horizontally, toasted

In a small saucepan simmer all ingredients except mushrooms and baguettes, stirring, until marinade is slightly reduced. Remove from heat and cool to room temperature. Add mushroom caps to saucepan and marinate, stirring occasionally, for one hour.

Preheat broiler. Drain mushrooms and arrange, stemmed sides up, on a broiler rack. Broil 2 inches from heat and turn over. Broil another 3–4 minutes or until tender. Transfer mushrooms to baguettes and top with Asian Coleslaw.

ASIAN COLESLAW:

2 tablespoons fat-free mayonnaise

1 tablespoon white vinegar

1 teaspoon toasted sesame oil*

1 teaspoon honey

1 cup finely shredded Napa cabbage

1 small carrot, finely shredded

¼ cup thinly sliced onion

In a medium bowl whisk together mayonnaise, vinegar, oil, and honey. Stir in remaining ingredients and mix well.

*See **Specialty Ingredients** (page 34)

NUTRIENT ANALYSIS PER SERVING:
Calories (kcal) 249.57

Protein (g) 7.89	Calories from Protein 31.10	% Calories from Protein 12.46
Carbohydrates(g) 47.48	Calories from Carbohydrates 187.10	% Calories from Carbohydrates 74.97
Fat (g) 3.54	Calories from Fat 31.37	% Calories from Fat 12.57
Saturated Fat (g) 0.65	Total Dietary Fiber (g) 3.73	Sodium (mg) 583.74

SANDWICHES OF ROSEMARY FIG CHUTNEY AND SMOKED CHICKEN BREAST

∞

*M*ake the chutney ahead of time, and these sandwiches are a snap to prepare. They're rich and smoky with a slightly sweet edge that's utterly irresistible. They pack beautifully for picnics or lunch at work.

MAKES 4 SERVINGS

1 lb. organic shaved smoked chicken breast
8 thick slices of rosemary sourdough bread, toasted
8 large fresh spinach leaves, washed, stems removed

CHUTNEY:

1 cup dried figs, finely chopped
½ cup red wine
½ cup water
¼ cup honey
2 teaspoons dried rosemary, crushed

In small heavy saucepan simmer all chutney ingredients over low heat, covered, for 30 minutes. Uncover and simmer, stirring frequently, until liquid evaporates and mixture thickens. Cool to room temperature. Assemble each sandwich with ¼ lb. smoked chicken, 2 tablespoon chutney, and 2 spinach leaves.

The chutney recipe makes about 1¼ cups, or ten 2-tablespoon servings. Chutney will keep in fridge for two months, or it may be frozen in an airtight container for up to 6 months.

NUTRIENT ANALYSIS PER SERVING SANDWICH WITHOUT CHUTNEY:
Calories (kcal) 382.23

Protein (g) 41.89	Calories from Protein 172.72	% Calories from Protein 45.19
Carbohydrates(g) 36.80	Calories from Carbohydrates 151.71	% Calories from Carbohydrates 39.69
Fat (g) 6.23	Calories from Fat 57.80	% Calories from Fat 15.12
Saturated Fat (g) 1.60	Cholesterol (mg) 96.39	Total Dietary Fiber (g) 2.65
Sodium (mg) 522.76		

NUTRIENT ANALYSIS PER SERVING OF CHUTNEY:
Calories (kcal) 83.21

Protein (g) 0.40	Calories from Protein 1.60	% Calories from Protein 1.92
Carbohydrates(g) 20.27	Calories from Carbohydrates 80.90	% Calories from Carbohydrates 97.22
Fat (g) 0.08	Calories from Fat 0.72	% Calories from Fat 0.86
Saturated Fat (g) 0.03	Total Dietary Fiber (g) 1.35	Sodium (mg) 1.46

SANDWICHES OF LEMON-HERB CHICKEN WITH WATERCRESS AND ROASTED RED PEPPERS
∞

These sandwiches have a wonderful, unusual combination of flavors whose sophistication belies their easy preparation. They are sure to be a lunchbox favorite.

MAKES 4 SERVINGS

2 organic skinless, boneless chicken breasts

2 tablespoons fresh lemon juice

2 tablespoons all-purpose unbleached white flour

1 teaspoon whole green peppercorns, crushed*

½ teaspoon rosemary, crushed

1 tablespoon olive oil

⅔ cup roasted red pepper strips **

1 medium bunch watercress, washed and spun dry, stems removed

8 thick slices of fresh sourdough bread, toasted

In a glass pie plate combine chicken with lemon juice and marinate for 10 minutes, turning once. In another pie plate stir together flour, crushed peppercorns, crushed rosemary, and salt to taste. Remove chicken from marinade, letting excess lemon juice drip off, and dredge in flour mixture. Reserve marinade.

In a large non-stick skillet heat oil over medium high heat and add chicken. Sauté for 3–4 minutes or until lightly browned. Turn chicken and cook another 5 minutes, or until cooked through. Remove chicken from skillet, let cool, and slice thinly. To skillet add reserved marinade, roasted pepper strips, and watercress, cooking just until liquid has evaporated and watercress wilts.

Assemble sandwiches with chicken, roasted pepper strips, and watercress.

*Green peppercorns are available in the spice section of grocery stores, or at spice shops.
**To roast red peppers, place whole peppers in broiler pan and broil as close to heat as possible, until skins are black and blistered, turning peppers occasionally so they char evenly. Let peppers cool, then slip off skins, remove stems, and seed. You can also roast peppers over a gas burner until blackened, then cool, skin, stem, and seed.

NUTRIENT ANALYSIS PER SERVING:
Calories (kcal) 267.54

Protein (g) 4.76	Calories from Protein 18.69	% Calories from Protein 6.98
Carbohydrates(g) 60.08	Calories from Carbohydrates 235.74	% Calories from Carbohydrates 88.11
Fat (g) 1.49	Calories from Fat 13.11	% Calories from Fat 4.90
Saturated Fat (g) 0.26	Total Dietary Fiber (g) 7.27	Sodium (mg) 343.34

SANDWICHES OF SWEET TOMATO-CURRANT CHUTNEY AND SMOKED TURKEY BREAST

∞

I love the chutney in this recipe—it livens up a typical turkey sandwich and turns it into something truly special.

MAKES 4 SERVINGS

 1 lb. organic shaved smoked turkey breast
 Small bunch fresh basil leaves, washed, stems removed

 Two 12" long narrow French bread baguettes, halved horizontally, toasted

CHUTNEY:

 14 oz. can whole tomatoes with juice
 ½ large onion, chopped
 Zest and juice of one lemon
 ¼ cup brown sugar
 1/4 cup apple cider vinegar

3 tablespoons raisins, chopped

1 teaspoon yellow mustard seeds

¼ teaspoon salt

⅛ teaspoon cayenne, or to taste

⅛ teaspoon ground allspice

⅛ teaspoon ground cinnamon

In a small heavy saucepan combine all chutney ingredients. Cook uncovered over medium low heat, stirring occasionally, 20 minutes. Reduce heat to low and simmer, stirring occasionally, for another 20 minutes, or until liquid evaporates and mixture thickens. Cool chutney to room temperature. Assemble each sandwich with ¼ lb. turkey, 2 tablespoons chutney, and several basil leaves.

The chutney recipe makes about 1¼ cups, or ten 2-tablespoon servings. It will keep chilled in an airtight container for up to 3 months.

NUTRIENT ANALYSIS PER SERVING SANDWICH WITHOUT CHUTNEY:

Calories (kcal) 343.81

Protein (g) 40.23	Calories from Protein 166.72	% Calories from Protein 48.49
Carbohydrates(g) 36.10	Calories from Carbohydrates 149.58	% Calories from Carbohydrates 43.51
Fat (g) 2.95	Calories from Fat 27.52	% Calories from Fat 8.00
Saturated Fat (g) 0.72	Cholesterol (mg) 94.12	Total Dietary Fiber (g) 2.11
Sodium (mg) 482.01		

NUTRIENT ANALYSIS PER SERVING OF CHUTNEY:

Calories (kcal) 34.19

Protein (g) 0.56	Calories from Protein 2.00	% Calories from Protein 5.84
Carbohydrates(g) 8.82	Calories from Carbohydrates 31.58	% Calories from Carbohydrates 92.37
Fat (g) 0.08	Calories from Fat 0.61	% Calories from Fat 1.79
Saturated Fat (g) 0.01	Total Dietary Fiber (g) 0.66	Sodium (mg) 64.18

ITALIAN LEMON TUNA SANDWICHES

∞

These sandwiches are my husband's creation, and they are a tangy, savory, safe alternative to the usual tuna salad which is loaded with fat. The lemon and basil are the key ingredients, and they give a delicious twist to this recipe.

MAKES 3 SERVINGS

3 tablespoons onion, finely chopped
1 medium garlic clove, minced
2 teaspoons extra-virgin olive oil
Juice of one lemon
1 teaspoon dried parsley
2 teaspoons dill weed
6 oz. can of solid white albacore tuna, packed in water, rinsed
Salt and pepper to taste
Small bunch fresh basil, stems removed, finely shredded
Small tomato, thinly sliced

One 18" long narrow French bread baguette, halved horizontally, toasted

Whisk the onion, garlic, oil, and lemon juice together, then whisk in parsley and dill. Stir in tuna until well blended, and season with salt and pepper to taste. Assemble sandwiches with fresh basil on the bottom, tuna in the middle, and tomato on top (this will keep the sandwiches from getting soggy).

NUTRIENT ANALYSIS PER SERVING:
Calories (kcal) 303.04

Protein (g) 19.99	Calories from Protein 80.72	% Calories from Protein 26.64
Carbohydrates(g) 39.49	Calories from Carbohydrates 159.47	% Calories from Carbohydrates 52.62
Fat (g) 6.92	Calories from Fat 62.85	% Calories from Fat 20.74
Saturated Fat (g) 1.32	Cholesterol (mg) 23.81	Total Dietary Fiber (g) 2.72
Sodium (mg) 640.22		

ENGLISH TEATIME SHRIMP AND WATERCRESS FINGER SANDWICHES

∞

I always think of these sandwiches as a special treat, even though the ingredients are ordinary and they are very fast and easy to make. They are especially delicious with an assortment of other finger foods, such as Sweet-Tart Orange Cranberry Bread (page 99), for a late afternoon meal.

MAKES 12 SMALL SANDWICHES, 3-4 SERVINGS

1 tablespoon whole green or white peppercorns
½ lb. shrimp, shelled and deveined
2 tablespoons soy cream cheese
2 tablespoons mango chutney*
Small bunch watercress, stems removed
12 small ½" thick slices of French or sourdough bread, toasted

Bring a small saucepan of water to boil and add peppercorns. Add shrimp and boil until just pink and cooked through, about 30–60 seconds. Drain. Halve shrimp horizontally.

Mix together soy cream cheese and mango chutney. Top toasted bread slices with chutney mixture, shrimp halves, and a few sprigs of watercress.

*Mango chutney is available in most grocery stores near the ketchup, or at specialty food stores or Indian markets.

NUTRIENT ANALYSIS PER SERVING:
Calories (kcal) 255.72

Protein (g) 21.23	Calories from Protein 86.78	% Calories from Protein 33.93
Carbohydrates(g) 33.73	Calories from Carbohydrates 137.89	% Calories from Carbohydrates 53.92
Fat (g) 3.38	Calories from Fat 31.05	% Calories from Fat 12.14
Saturated Fat (g) 0.66	Cholesterol (mg) 114.84	Total Dietary Fiber (g) 2.23
Sodium (mg) 486.76		

LOUISIANA BARBECUED CATFISH SANDWICHES WITH SWEET AND SOUR WILTED CABBAGE SLAW

∞

*S*erve these sandwiches topped with the slaw, a handful of baked potato chips on the side, and a cool herbal ice tea, and you've got the perfect backyard barbecue meal.

MAKES 4 SANDWICHES

1½ pounds catfish fillets
¼ cup bourbon
¼ cup soy sauce
¼ cup whole grain mustard
¼ cup ketchup
¼ cup packed brown sugar
1½ teaspoons dried rosemary, crushed
¼ teaspoon cumin

Two 12" long narrow French bread baguettes, halved horizontally, toasted

Rinse and dry the catfish fillets and set aside. In a small bowl combine remaining ingredients (except bread), and microwave on high for 5 minutes, or until slightly reduced. Coat catfish with ½ cup barbecue sauce. Heat a large non-stick skillet over medium heat, spray with cooking oil, and sauté catfish until golden brown on both sides until cooked through.

Halve baguettes horizontally and toast lightly. Top with catfish, remaining barbecue sauce, and wilted slaw to form sandwiches.

SWEET AND SOUR WILTED CABBAGE SLAW

1½ cups finely shredded green cabbage
1½ cups finely shredded red cabbage
1 small carrot, finely shredded
½ small onion, thinly sliced
¼ cup apple cider vinegar
2 teaspoons granulated sugar
½ teaspoon celery seed, crushed

In a small bowl stir together vinegar, sugar, and celery seed until sugar dissolves. In a large non-stick skillet sprayed with cooking oil sauté onion until softened. Add cabbage and carrot and cook over medium low heat, stirring frequently, until just tender. Add vinegar mixture and salt and pepper to taste.

NUTRIENT ANALYSIS PER SERVING:
Calories (kcal) 446.05

Protein (g) 36.25	Calories from Protein 145.11	% Calories from Protein 32.53
Carbohydrates(g) 58.99	Calories from Carbohydrates 236.15	% Calories from Carbohydrates 52.94
Fat (g) 7.19	Calories from Fat 64.79	% Calories from Fat 14.52
Saturated Fat (g) 1.71	Cholesterol (mg) 98.66	Total Dietary Fiber (g) 4.50
Sodium (mg) 1225.64		

OPEN-FACE CHESAPEAKE CRAB CAKE SANDWICHES

∞

*C*rab cakes are so delicious, but almost every restaurant serves them deep-fried. There's no need! These delectable little sandwiches can be baked or even pan-fried to a golden, crispy brown and still be perfectly safe. So splurge on some fresh crab meat and give yourself a tasty treat.

MAKES 6-8 SMALL SANDWICHES

½ cup finely diced onion
½ cup finely diced celery
1 tablespoon canola oil
12 oz. lump crab meat
⅓ cup fine dry bread crumbs
½ cup fat-free mayonnaise
1½ teaspoons Old Bay seasoning*
½ teaspoon Worcestershire sauce
1 teaspoon dijon mustard

6–8 small slices of sourdough bread, toasted
Lemon wedges for serving

Preheat oven to 350°F. In a large non-stick skillet cook onion and celery in oil over medium low heat until tender. Transfer to a medium bowl, and add remaining ingredients, folding together gently but thoroughly. With an ice cream scoop or a ¼ cup-measuring cup, form small mounds of crab cake mixture on a cookie sheet sprayed with cooking oil. Bake for 25 minutes or until golden brown. Top each toast slice with a crab cake and serve each sandwich with a lemon wedge.

*Old Bay seasoning is available at many grocery stores, fish markets, and specialty foods shops.

NUTRIENT ANALYSIS PER SERVING:
Calories (kcal) 161.30

Protein (g) 14.36	Calories from Protein 58.73	% Calories from Protein 36.41
Carbohydrates(g) 16.07	Calories from Carbohydrates 65.74	% Calories from Carbohydrates 40.76
Fat (g) 4.00	Calories from Fat 36.82	% Calories from Fat 22.83
Saturated Fat (g) 0.52	Cholesterol (mg) 50.43	Total Dietary Fiber (g) 1.10
Sodium (mg) 760.37		

TOASTED BAGELS WITH LOX AND LEMON-CAPER CREAM CHEESE

∞

*B*agels are a wonderful IBS staple, and lox has to be their most luxurious accompaniment. I can't think of a better combination of flavors than in this recipe, so enjoy.

MAKES 2 SANDWICH HALVES, 1-2 SERVINGS

- 1 tablespoon soy cream cheese
- 1 tablespoon capers, chopped
- ½ teaspoon freshly grated lemon zest
- 1 plain bagel, halved, toasted
- 4 oz. lox or other smoked salmon
- Two thin slices of red onion

Combine soy cream cheese, capers, and zest. Top bagel halves evenly with cream cheese mixture, lox, and red onion. Serve open-faced.

NUTRIENT ANALYSIS PER SERVING:

Calories (kcal) 388.94

Protein (g) 30.83	Calories from Protein 125.97	% Calories from Protein 32.39
Carbohydrates(g) 49.26	Calories from Carbohydrates 201.31	% Calories from Carbohydrates 51.76
Fat (g) 6.71	Calories from Fat 61.66	% Calories from Fat 15.85
Saturated Fat (g) 1.31	Cholesterol (mg) 26.07	Total Dietary Fiber (g) 2.74
Sodium (mg) 2999.03		

PUMPERNICKEL BAGELS
WITH SMOKED TROUT
AND DILLED CUCUMBERS
∞

*S*moked fish is a great safe substitute for lunch meats and cheeses. It's low fat, high protein, and above all delicious! Combined with dill and cucumber it makes a gourmet sandwich in no time flat.

MAKES 2 SANDWICH HALVES, 1-2 SERVINGS

8 thin cucumber slices
½ teaspoon dill weed
1 pumpernickel bagel, halved, toasted
1 tablespoon soy cream cheese
4 oz. smoked trout or other white fish

Toss cucumber slices with dill. Top bagel halves with soy cream cheese, dilled cucumbers, and smoked trout. Serve open face.

NUTRIENT ANALYSIS PER SERVING:
Calories (kcal) 379.02
Protein (g) 36.64
Carbohydrates(g) 49.40
Fat (g) 2.85
Saturated Fat (g) 0.51
Sodium (mg) 1634.24

Calories from Protein 150.22
Calories from Carbohydrates 202.55
Calories from Fat 26.25
Cholesterol (mg) 37.40

% Calories from Protein 39.63
% Calories from Carbohydrates 53.44
% Calories from Fat 6.93
Total Dietary Fiber (g) 2.67

MAIN DISHES

∞

*D*INNER'S ON! WOULDN'T it be great if you could safely eat it? Well, here's terrific news—with these recipes, you finally can. Many people are already in the habit of having a soluble fiber base with their dinners, whether pasta, potatoes, rice, or bread. It's very easy to work from this foundation to create delicious meals while keeping just a few other considerations in mind. Simple substitutions of seafood or chicken breasts for meat, soy milk for dairy, and the use of low fat cooking techniques will quickly give you safe dinners with no extra effort. Just remember that main dishes should incorporate as many fresh vegetables as possible, and beans or nuts make healthy additions as well.

There are so many delicious dinner choices to look forward to, from traditional homestyle favorites to exciting ethnic specialties, that the only difficulty you'll likely face is choosing just one to eat tonight. You have many wonderful, healthy meals ahead of you—enjoy!

ITALIAN CROSTINI WITH HONEY-TOMATO SAUCE AND GARLIC SAFFRON PRAWNS

∞

*T*his recipe has been a favorite since the day I created it over ten years ago. It has a fabulous combination of flavors—toasty fresh bread, subtly sweet and cumin-scented tomato sauce, and intensely garlic-flavored prawns. The colors of this dish are beautiful as well—the saffron tints the prawns a brilliant yellow against the scarlet sauce.

The longer you simmer the tomatoes the better—the liquid will reduce and the flavors will mellow and richen. Leftover sauce and prawns are easily frozen and very handy to have in the freezer for a 5–minute dinner.

MAKES 3-4 SERVINGS

PRAWNS:

1 cup water
6 large garlic cloves, minced
Dash salt
⅛ teaspoon saffron threads
1 lb. medium prawns, shelled and deveined

Bring water to boil in small saucepan with garlic, salt, and saffron. Add prawns and simmer just until pink and curled. Reserve ¼ cup cooking liquid and drain prawns. Slice each prawn in half lengthwise.

SAUCE:

3 large ripe tomatoes, diced
1 small onion, diced
3 large cloves garlic, minced
1½ tablespoons honey
1 teaspoon olive oil
¼ teaspoon ground cumin
⅛ teaspoon cayenne pepper, or to taste
¼ cup reserved prawn cooking liquid

Combine all sauce ingredients in medium saucepan. Bring to a boil, reduce heat and simmer about 45 minutes, until thickened. Purée the sauce in a blender.

CROSTINI:

French or Sourdough bread baguette, sliced into 1" slices
2 tablespoons soy Parmesan or Romano cheese

Place bread slices on cookie sheet and broil until golden. Turn slices over and broil other side. Top with the saffron sauce, prawn halves, and a light sprinkle of Parmesan or Romano. Return to broiler until cheese slightly melts. Serve immediately.

NUTRIENT ANALYSIS PER SERVING:
Calories (kcal) 553.56

Protein (g) 36.93	Calories from Protein 148.34	% Calories from Protein 26.80
Carbohydrates (g) 82.55	Calories from Carbohydrates 331.61	% Calories from Carbohydrates 59.91
Fat (g) 8.14	Calories from Fat 73.61	% Calories from Fat 13.30
Saturated Fat (g) 1.87	Cholesterol (mg) 174.34	Total Dietary Fiber (g) 5.77
Sodium (mg) 1027.55		

TANDOORI SPICED MANGO SHRIMP
∞

*T*his is a wonderful Indian-inspired meal, spicy but not hot. The mango and lime add a sweet and tangy flair, and the basmati rice provides a deliciously nutty base.

MAKES 3-4 SERVINGS

1 lb. shrimp, shelled and deveined
¼ cup chopped fresh cilantro
1 tablespoon canola oil

Fresh basmati rice for serving (see page 126)

SAUCE:

3 tablespoons mango chutney*
¼ cup fresh lime juice
Dash cayenne pepper (optional)

Force chutney through a sieve into a bowl and whisk in lime juice and dash of cayenne. Set aside.

TANDOORI SPICE PASTE:

1½ teaspoons paprika
1 teaspoon ground cumin
1 teaspoon ground coriander
4 garlic cloves, minced
1" piece fresh gingerroot, minced
Zest of one lime
Juice of one lime

In a large skillet dry-roast paprika, cumin, and coriander over medium heat, stirring occasionally, until spices are several shades darker and fragrant, about 4 minutes. Combine spices and all remaining spice paste ingredients in a medium bowl. Add shrimp, stirring well to evenly coat. Marinate for 20–30 minutes.

Heat oil in a large non-stick skillet over medium high heat and add shrimp, sautée-ing until golden and just cooked through. Serve over basmati rice and top with cilantro and sauce.

*Mango chutney is available in most grocery stores near the ketchup, or at specialty food stores or Indian markets.

NUTRIENT ANALYSIS PER SERVING:
Calories (kcal) 218.10

Protein (g) 30.99	Calories from Protein 125.54	% Calories from Protein 57.56
Carbohydrates(g) 6.28	Calories from Carbohydrates 25.46	% Calories from Carbohydrates 11.67
Fat (g) 7.36	Calories from Fat 67.10	% Calories from Fat 30.77
Saturated Fat (g) 0.84	Cholesterol (mg) 229.82	Total Dietary Fiber (g) 0.43
Sodium (mg) 226.38		

MEXICAN SAUTÉED PEPITAS PRAWNS

*T*his dish has an earthy, haunting flavor that comes from the toasted pumpkin seeds, which are finely ground to make their insoluble fiber tolerable.

MAKES 4 SERVINGS

I lb. prawns, rinsed, shelled, and deveined, coarsely chopped
½ cup green pumpkin seeds (pepitas)*
½ teaspoon coriander seeds
I small onion, diced
4 garlic cloves, mashed
I large tomato, diced
I small red bell pepper, roasted**
¼ teaspoon salt
Dash cayenne pepper (optional)
3 teaspoons olive oil, divided
Juice of one lime
I cup finely chopped fresh cilantro

Baked corn chips (Tostitos), flour tortillas, or rice for serving

Toast the pumpkin seeds in a large, ungreased (not non-stick) frying pan over medium high heat until they crackle, shaking pan constantly. Do not brown. Cool. Add the pumpkin seeds and the coriander seeds to a food processor or blender and grind to a fine powder. Add the onion, garlic, tomato, roasted red pepper, salt, cayenne, and 2 teaspoons olive oil. Puree until smooth. Pour the sauce into a small saucepan and simmer, covered, over medium low heat for 20–30 minutes to mellow flavors. Add salt and pepper to taste, and cayenne if desired.

Heat 1 teaspoon olive oil in a large non-stick skillet over medium high heat. Add the chopped prawns and sauté until they just begin to turn pink. Stir the sauce into the skillet and heat through until shrimp are cooked. Remove from heat and stir in the lime juice and cilantro. Serve with chips, flour tortillas, or over rice.

*See **Specialty Ingredients** (page 34)

**To roast red peppers, place whole peppers in broiler pan and broil as close to heat as possible, until skins are black and blistered, turning peppers occasionally so they char evenly. Let peppers cool, then slip off skins, remove stems, and seed. Or roast peppers over a gas burner until evenly charred, then cool and remove skins, stems, and seeds.

NUTRIENT ANALYSIS PER SERVING:
Calories (kcal) 216.71

Protein (g) 25.74	Calories from Protein 102.55	% Calories from Protein 47.32
Carbohydrates(g) 12.49	Calories from Carbohydrates 49.77	% Calories from Carbohydrates 22.97
Fat (g) 7.18	Calories from Fat 64.39	% Calories from Fat 29.71
Saturated Fat (g) 1.16	Cholesterol (mg) 172.37	Total Dietary Fiber (g) 1.92
Sodium (mg) 326.42		

THAI-FRIED RICE
WITH CILANTRO AND SHRIMP
∞

*M*y husband created this very low fat fried rice, and oh, how I love it! The prep work is a little time-consuming, but it cooks very quickly, and makes a terrifically delicious and completely nutritious meal all by itself. It keeps and reheats beautifully, and is a staple of mine for work lunches. Make sure you have plenty of lime wedges—they add the perfect tangy note to the smoky flavors of the rice.

MAKES 6-8 SERVINGS

4 cups cold cooked jasmine rice
8 large cloves garlic
½ cup packed fresh chopped cilantro
2 tablespoons canola oil
I cup diced onion
I cup diced carrots
¾ lb. shelled and deveined raw shrimp
3 organic egg whites
¼ cup Thai or Vietnamese fish sauce*
3 tablespoons Mushroom Soy Sauce
I tablespoon brown sugar
½ teaspoon white pepper
2 scallions, diced
I cup fresh or frozen green peas

Lime wedges for serving

Knead the cold rice gently through your fingers to separate the grains (rinse your hands in cold water first so the rice doesn't stick). Set aside.

Blend the garlic and cilantro to a paste in a food processor. Place all ingredients within easy reach of the stove.

Set a wok over medium-high heat. When it's very hot, add the oil, tilting wok to coat sides. When the oil is hot, add the garlic-cilantro paste, onion, and carrot, and fry until the onion is transparent. Add the shrimp and fry just until they begin to turn pink. Add egg whites, stirring them at the bottom of the wok until cooked, then mix them in to the other ingredients.

Add the rice and stir well, then press the rice mixture into the bottom of the wok to fry for several minutes. Turn the mixture over, stir, and press down into the wok again. While rice is cooking, stir together fish sauce, soy sauce, sugar, and white pepper. Add the liquid down the sides of the wok, and stir well, and fry for 2–3 minutes. Add the scallions and peas, stir well and fry just until the scallions are limp.

Serve fried rice with wedges of fresh lime.

*See **Specialty Ingredients** (page 34)

NUTRIENT ANALYSIS PER SERVING:
Calories (kcal) 303.64

Protein (g) 19.23	Calories from Protein 78.05	% Calories from Protein 25.70
Carbohydrates(g) 41.75	Calories from Carbohydrates 169.42	% Calories from Carbohydrates 55.80
Fat (g) 6.15	Calories from Fat 56.17	% Calories from Fat 18.50
Saturated Fat (g) 0.63	Cholesterol (mg) 86.18	Total Dietary Fiber (g) 2.84
Sodium (mg) 1377.25		

SIZZLING SHRIMP FAJITAS WITH BAJA ORANGE MARINADE

∞

These fajitas make a regular appearance in my kitchen, because they are fast, easy, delicious, and dependably safe. This is a great recipe to serve to guests, as everyone can customize their fajitas with whatever fillings suit their fancy. Serve a big bowl of baked corn chips with the extra salsas and dips, and you'll have a Mexican fiesta!

MAKES 6 SERVINGS

1½ lbs. shelled and deveined raw shrimp (or red snapper, catfish, or rock cod)

Make a marinade by stirring together in a glass pie plate:
¼ cup fresh lime juice
¼ cup fresh orange juice
1 tablespoon olive oil
4 minced garlic cloves
1 teaspoon ground chipotle pepper*
2 tablespoons minced fresh cilantro

Fresh flour tortillas for serving

Add shrimp (or fish) and marinate for 20 minutes. Remove shrimp from marinade and grill or broil just until cooked through, turning once. Shrimp will cook more quickly than fish, approximately 2 minutes per side. Exact time for fish will depend on the thickness of the fillets—typically, 10 minutes per inch, total. Serve on fresh flour tortillas, and allow each person to customize their fajitas with the following:

Shredded cabbage
Diced onion
Fresh chopped cilantro
Smoky Black Bean Dip (page 54)
Tex-Mex Guacamole (page 63)
Sweet Mango and Roasted Tomato Salsa (page 67)

Serve baked corn chips (Tostitos) as accompaniment.

*See **Specialty Ingredients** (page 34)

NUTRIENT ANALYSIS PER SERVING OF SHRIMP FAJITA FILLING:

Calories (kcal) 150.68

Protein (g) 23.29	Calories from Protein 95.91	% Calories from Protein 63.65
Carbohydrates(g) 3.73	Calories from Carbohydrates 15.34	% Calories from Carbohydrates 10.18
Fat (g) 4.26	Calories from Fat 39.44	% Calories from Fat 26.17
Saturated Fat (g) 0.68	Cholesterol (mg) 172.37	Total Dietary Fiber (g) 0.13
Sodium (mg) 168.81		

BARBECUED VIETNAMESE CALAMARI WITH SWEET AND TANGY DIPPING SAUCE

∞

his recipe is fast, simple, and utterly delicious. If you've never had calamari before this is the perfect recipe for your first try. The sweet chili sauce is a wonderful accompaniment to the mild, slightly chewy yet smoky-tender grilled squid.

MAKES **4** SERVINGS

> 2 lbs. fresh cleaned squid steaks, cut lengthwise into 2" wide strips
> About 20 bamboo or metal skewers (if bamboo, soak in cold water for an hour before using)
>
> Cooked jasmine rice for serving (see page 126)

Thread the squid strips onto the skewers, keeping the strips as extended as possible so they lie flat. Grill over a charcoal barbecue or stove grill, turning once, for about 5 minutes total. The squid should turn opaque and firm but still be tender. Serve over jasmine rice with dipping sauce and Asian Sweet Pickled Cucumbers (page 123).

SWEET AND TANGY DIPPING SAUCE:

> ¼ cup white vinegar
> ½ cup granulated sugar
> ¼ teaspoon salt
> 2 teaspoons chili garlic paste*

Add all ingredients except chili garlic paste to a small saucepan. Bring to a boil over high heat, then reduce heat to low and simmer, stirring, until mixture reduces and thickens to a syrup. Remove from heat and add the chili garlic paste. Let cool to room temperature.

*See **Specialty Ingredients** (page 34)

NUTRIENT ANALYSIS PER SERVING WITH SAUCE:
Calories (kcal) 307.51

Protein (g) 35.34	Calories from Protein 144.45	% Calories from Protein 46.97
Carbohydrates (g) 32.85	Calories from Carbohydrates 134.27	% Calories from Carbohydrates 43.66
Fat (g) 3.13	Calories from Fat 28.79	% Calories from Fat 9.36
Saturated Fat (g) 0.81	Cholesterol (mg) 528.44	Sodium (mg) 245.53

JILL'S CHILEAN SEA BASS GLAZED WITH CRANBERRY SAUCE

∾

*T*his recipe is courtesy of Jill Sklar, a fabulous friend and cook. She likes it with steamed aspara- gus, and so do I. It is also wonderful with Simple Sweet Cornbread (page 113) or Old- Fashioned Bread Stuffing with Dried Apricots and Currants (page 130).

MAKES 4-6 SERVINGS

2 pounds Chilean sea bass fillets
2 tablespoons olive oil
Half a ripe lemon

CRANBERRY SAUCE:

One 16 oz. package of fresh cranberries
1 cup granulated sugar
1 tablespoon lemon zest

Preheat oven to 400°F. Rinse the fish with fresh water and pat dry. Place it in a shal- low, oven-proof baking dish and rub with the oil. Cook the fish, uncovered, for 15 min- utes, then remove from oven and squeeze the lemon over the fish. Return to oven and cook another 10 minutes, or until the juices run clear and the fish flakes when a fork is inserted into the center of the fillet.

While the fish cooks, add the cranberry sauce ingredients to a small saucepan. Bring mixture to a boil, reduce heat, and simmer until all the cranberries pop. Force mixture through a sieve and discard skins and seeds. Top the fish with the cranberry sauce to serve.

NUTRIENT ANALYSIS PER SERVING:

Calories (kcal) 352.49

Protein (g) 28.16	Calories from Protein 112.39	% Calories from Protein 31.89
Carbohydrates (g) 42.89	Calories from Carbohydrates 171.17	% Calories from Carbohydrates 48.56
Fat (g) 7.68	Calories from Fat 68.93	% Calories from Fat 19.55
Saturated Fat (g) 1.39	Cholesterol (mg) 61.99	Total Dietary Fiber (g) 3.18
Sodium (mg) 103.91		

BROILED RED SNAPPER WITH PIQUANT TAMARIND GLAZE

∞

*H*ere's a fast and easy way to make a delicious fish dinner. The tamarind glaze adds a fantastic sweet and sour tang—be sure and serve it with lots of rice to catch every last drop.

MAKES **4** SERVINGS

- I cup water
- 2 tablespoons TamCon tamarind concentrate*
- 6 cloves garlic, minced
- 2 tablespoons Thai or Vietnamese fish sauce*
- I tablespoon honey
- I tablespoon finely chopped cilantro
- 4 six-ounce red snapper fillets
- 2 scallions, finely diced
- 2 tablespoons finely shredded fresh basil

Jasmine rice for serving (see page 126)

In a medium bowl combine first 6 ingredients and microwave on high about 8–9 minutes, until sauce has reduced to one cup. Season fish fillets with salt and pepper, and broil 4–5 inches from heat until just cooked through, about 7–8 minutes. Transfer fish to serving platter and top with sauce, scallions, and basil. Serve with rice.

*See **Specialty Ingredients** (page 34)

NUTRIENT ANALYSIS PER SERVING:
Calories (kcal) 265.58

Protein (g) 47.61	Calories from Protein 197.54	% Calories from Protein 74.38
Carbohydrates(g) 9.40	Calories from Carbohydrates 39.01	% Calories from Carbohydrates 14.69
Fat (g) 3.11	Calories from Fat 29.03	% Calories from Fat 10.93
Saturated Fat (g) 0.66	Cholesterol (mg) 83.92	Total Dietary Fiber (g) 0.62
Sodium (mg) 843.98		

MUSTARD DILL SALMON WITH ROASTED POTATOES AND GREENS

*T*his is a wonderfully hearty and filling dinner, with a terrific combination of flavors. Salmon and dill are a classic match, and the high soluble fiber base of potatoes allows for the addition of fresh greens. The rich and tangy mustard glaze gives a delicate golden sheen to the whole dish.

MAKES 4 SERVINGS

⅓ cup dijon mustard
1 tablespoon canola oil
1 tablespoon dill weed
4 tablespoons packed brown sugar
1½ pounds new potatoes, cut into ¼" slices
1 lb. salmon fillet
1 small bunch mustard or spinach greens, stems removed, roughly chopped

Preheat oven to 350°F. Mix mustard, oil, dill, and brown sugar in a small bowl. Place sliced potatoes in a large bowl and drizzle with ¼ cup of mustard sauce. Toss until evenly coated. Arrange potatoes in a single layer in a 9 x 13" baking pan sprayed with cooking oil. Bake 35 minutes.

Remove pan from oven and push potatoes to one side of pan. Place salmon fillet in center of pan and top with 1 tablespoon mustard sauce. Bake, uncovered, until salmon is just cooked through and potatoes are golden and tender, about 20–25 minutes.

While the salmon bakes, place greens in a large non-stick skillet. Toss with 2 tablespoons mustard sauce and sauté over medium high heat until greens are wilted, about 4–5 minutes. Divide greens among three plates, and top with baked salmon and potatoes. Top with remaining sauce.

NUTRIENT ANALYSIS PER SERVING:

Calories (kcal) 460.43

Protein (g) 28.20	Calories from Protein 112.34	% Calories from Protein 24.40
Carbohydrates(g) 52.22	Calories from Carbohydrates 208.05	% Calories from Carbohydrates 45.19
Fat (g) 15.62	Calories from Fat 140.03	% Calories from Fat 30.41
Saturated Fat (g) 3.15	Cholesterol (mg) 74.84	Total Dietary Fiber (g) 4.55
Sodium (mg) 77.94		

MAPLE-GLAZED SALMON WITH NUTTY WHEAT BERRIES

∞

ere is a recipe that is just as beautiful as is delicious. If you've never had wheat berries before you're in for a treat—they're nutty, chewy, and perfect with the salmon. The maple glaze and pecans add a delectable combination of flavors. See if this doesn't become one of your favorite meals.

MAKES 3 SERVINGS

5 tablespoons pure maple syrup
3 tablespoons soy sauce
¼ cup fresh lemon juice
1 tablespoon Dijon mustard
2 tablespoons olive oil
3½ cups water
½ cup wheat berries*
½ teaspoon salt
¼ cup diced scallions
12 ounce salmon fillet, cut into two or three portions
½ cup pecans, chopped
1 cup mesclun

In a small bowl whisk together first 4 ingredients, then slowly whisk in oil. Set vinaigrette aside.

In a small saucepan bring water, wheat berries, and salt to a boil, reduce heat and simmer, uncovered, for 45 minutes to 1 hour, until wheat berries are tender (add additional water as necessary to keep berries covered while cooking). Drain. In a medium bowl stir together ¼ cup vinaigrette, wheat berries, and green onion. Spoon mixture onto serving plates and set aside.

Heat a large non-stick skillet over medium heat and add pecans, stirring until toasted. Transfer pecans to a small bowl but don't wash skillet.

Rinse and dry salmon. Heat skillet over medium heat and spray with cooking oil. Add salmon and cook until golden brown, about 4–5 minutes. Turn salmon over and cook about 4–5 minutes more, or until just cooked through. Top wheat berry mixture with cooked salmon, drizzle with remaining vinaigrette, and sprinkle with toasted pecans and mesclun.

*Wheat berries are available in the bulk section of health food stores, specialty food shops, or see Directory of Resources.

NUTRIENT ANALYSIS PER SERVING:

Calories (kcal) 515.42		
Protein (g) 28.19	Calories from Protein 107.96	% Calories from Protein 20.95
Carbohydrates(g) 35.79	Calories from Carbohydrates 137.06	% Calories from Carbohydrates 26.59
Fat (g) 31.38	Calories from Fat 270.39	% Calories from Fat 52.46
Saturated Fat (g) 3.96	Cholesterol (mg) 70.27	Total Dietary Fiber (g) 5.94
Sodium (mg) 1045.65		

TEDDY'S HONEY MESQUITE SALMON
∞

*T*his is a very mild, subtly seasoned recipe. Mesquite smoke powder lends a slightly spicy, smoky accent that is delicious with the salmon.

MAKES 4 SERVINGS

 1 lb. salmon fillet
 Juice of half a lemon
 1 tablespoon honey
 ¾ teaspoon mesquite smoke powder*

Place salmon in a large baking pan. Combine remaining ingredients in a small bowl. Pour over salmon. Marinate for 20–30 minutes.

Preheat oven to 350°F. Bake salmon, uncovered, for 15–20 minutes, until fish just flakes.

*Mesquite smoke powder is available in the barbecue sauce section of some grocery stores, at spice shops, or see the Directory of Resources.

NUTRIENT ANALYSIS PER SERVING:

Calories (kcal) 207.94		
Protein (g) 24.19	Calories from Protein 98.90	% Calories from Protein 47.56
Carbohydrates(g) 4.83	Calories from Carbohydrates 19.76	% Calories from Carbohydrates 9.50
Fat (g) 9.71	Calories from Fat 89.29	% Calories from Fat 42.94
Saturated Fat (g) 1.70	Cholesterol (mg) 70.31	Total Dietary Fiber (g) 0.03
Sodium (mg) 53.57		

WOK-STEAMED TERIYAKI GINGER SALMON

∾

*W*hen you don't have much time to cook this is a fast and easy way to make a safe, nutri-tious dinner. What a bonus that it's incredibly delicious as well! Serve this with *Asian Sweet Pickled Cucumbers* (page 123) or *Steamed Sweet Potatoes with Japanese Miso Dressing* (page 121) for a fabulous meal.

MAKES 6 SERVINGS

1½ lbs. fresh salmon fillets
One small bunch green onions, cleaned
⅓ cup fresh gingerroot sliced into thin coins

Fresh rose rice for serving (see page 125)

TERIYAKI SAUCE:

¼ cup soy sauce
2 tablespoons mirin*
3 tablespoons white vinegar
1 tablespoon minced peeled fresh gingerroot
2 minced garlic cloves
2 tablespoons honey

Combine all teriyaki ingredients in a small bowl and set aside.

Place fish fillets on top of scallions on a steamer tray and sprinkle with the ginger coins. Steam covered, until fish flakes, about 8 minutes. Transfer to serving platter, dis-card scallions and ginger. Top with spoonfuls of teriyaki sauce and serve with rice.

*See **Specialty Ingredients** (page 34)

NUTRIENT ANALYSIS PER SERVING:
Calories (kcal) 220.69

Protein (g) 24.86	Calories from Protein 101.05	% Calories from Protein 45.79
Carbohydrates(g) 7.56	Calories from Carbohydrates 30.74	% Calories from Carbohydrates 13.93
Fat (g) 9.72	Calories from Fat 88.91	% Calories from Fat 40.29
Saturated Fat (g) 1.70	Cholesterol (mg) 70.31	Total Dietary Fiber (g) 0.13
Sodium (mg) 453.78		

HERBED PARMESAN-CRUSTED BAY SCALLOPS

∞

This is a simple yet sophisticated classic seafood recipe.

MAKES 4 SERVINGS

1½ lbs. bay scallops
1 tablespoon olive oil
2 garlic cloves, minced
1 large shallot, minced
¼ teaspoon garlic salt
Freshly ground black pepper to taste
2 tablespoons fresh parsley, finely chopped
½ cup fresh bread crumbs
¼ cup soy Parmesan

Fresh crusty French bread for serving

Bring a small saucepan full of water to boil, add scallops, and cook for 2 minutes. Drain well. Heat oil in a small non-stick skillet and fry the garlic and shallot over medium heat until tender. Add the scallops, salt, pepper, and parsley. Transfer mixture to 9″ baking pan, and sprinkle with bread crumbs and Parmesan. Place under broiler until golden brown and hot. Serve with fresh crusty French bread.

NUTRIENT ANALYSIS PER SERVING:
Calories (kcal) 236.88

Protein (g) 30.39	Calories from Protein 125.69	% Calories from Protein 53.06
Carbohydrates(g) 14.72	Calories from Carbohydrates 60.88	% Calories from Carbohydrates 25.70
Fat (g) 5.41	Calories from Fat 50.32	% Calories from Fat 21.24
Saturated Fat (g) 0.76	Cholesterol (mg) 56.13	Total Dietary Fiber (g)* 0.36
Sodium (mg) 536.13		

CORNMEAL-CRUSTED CAJUN CATFISH

∽

*S*erve these *"I-can't-believe-they're-not-fried"* fish fillets with Candied Sweet Potatoes (page 119) and fresh crusty French bread for a casual and delicious Southern-style meal.

MAKES 4 SERVINGS

1½ lbs. catfish fillets, rinsed and dried
⅓ cup yellow cornmeal
2 teaspoons Cajun seasoning (or substitute Old Bay seasoning), or to taste

French bread for serving
Fresh lemon wedges for serving

Combine Cajun seasoning and cornmeal in a large pie plate. Coat the catfish fillets evenly on all sides with the cornmeal mixture. Heat a large non-stick skillet over medium heat, spray pan with cooking oil, and cook catfish until golden brown and crispy on both sides and cooked through at the center. Squeeze lemon wedges over fish and serve.

Cᴀᴊᴜɴ Sᴇᴀsᴏɴɪɴɢ:

3 tablespoons sweet paprika

2 teaspoons garlic powder

2 teaspoons garlic salt

1 teaspoon white pepper

1 teaspoon black pepper

1 teaspoon chili powder

1 teaspoon basil, crushed

1 teaspoon thyme, crushed

½ teaspoon rosemary, crushed

Mix all ingredients together well and transfer to an airtight container for storage. Makes about ⅓ cup.

Nᴜᴛʀɪᴇɴᴛ Aɴᴀʟʏsɪs Pᴇʀ Sᴇʀᴠɪɴɢ:
Calories (kcal) 203.69
Protein (g) 28.84
Carbohydrates(g) 8.93
Fat (g) 4.99
Saturated Fat (g) 1.25
Sodium (mg) 112.25

Calories from Protein 119.90
Calories from Carbohydrates 37.14
Calories from Fat 46.65
Cholesterol (mg) 98.66

% Calories from Protein 58.86
% Calories from Carbohydrates 18.23
% Calories from Fat 22.90
Total Dietary Fiber (g) 0.85

CARAMELIZED SCALLOPS WITH GARLIC CHAMPAGNE GLAZE

∞

*T*his is an unusual dish with a sweet, tangy, and garlicky combination of flavors. Scallops are a great seafood staple for IBS because they're so low fat, and with delicious recipes like this one they're a perfectly safe indulgence.

MAKES 4 SERVINGS

1 tablespoon olive oil

1 lb. bay or sea scallops

4 large garlic cloves, minced

¼ cup maple syrup

¼ cup apple cider

¼ cup Champagne or white wine

3 tablespoons chopped shallots

¼ teaspoon dill weed

⅛ teaspoon salt

In a large heavy frying pan heat olive oil until hot but not smoking, and sauté scallops until golden on each side. Remove scallops from pan and keep warm. Add to pan garlic, syrup, and apple cider. Bring to a boil and cook until liquid is reduced to a glaze, about 3 minutes. Add remaining ingredients and boil until liquid reduces, about 4 minutes. Add scallops and cook just until they are heated through. Serve immediately.

NUTRIENT ANALYSIS PER SERVING:
Calories (kcal) 216.95

Protein (g) 19.45	Calories from Protein 84.83	% Calories from Protein 39.10
Carbohydrates(g) 20.57	Calories from Carbohydrates 89.75	% Calories from Carbohydrates 41.37
Fat (g) 4.32	Calories from Fat 42.36	% Calories from Fat 19.53
Saturated Fat (g) 0.56	Cholesterol (mg) 37.42	Total Dietary Fiber (g)* 0.08
Sodium (mg) 260.22		

SEARED FRESH TUNA STEAKS WITH CRUSHED CORIANDER AND CITRUS MISO SAUCE

*F*resh tuna is a real treat, especially for meat-lovers. It is probably the heartiest fish, and should be cooked until just barely done at the center or it will be dry. Giving it a spice rub and then searing it is a delectable way to treat tuna, and because it is so flavorful it can stand up to an assertive sauce like the citrus miso.

MAKES 6 SERVINGS

6 six ounce tuna steaks
3 tablespoons whole coriander seeds, crushed with a mortar and pestle

SAUCE:

¼ cup miso paste*
¼ cup fresh lemon juice
¼ cup fresh orange juice
2 teaspoons white vinegar
3 tablespoons mirin*
2 tablespoons granulated sugar
½ teaspoon Japanese soy sauce (such as Kikkoman)

Fresh jasmine rice for serving (see page 126)

In a shallow pan coat the tuna steaks with the crushed coriander seeds. Stir together sauce ingredients and set aside.

In non-stick frying pan sprayed with cooking oil, sear tuna steaks over medium high heat for 3–5 minutes per side, until pink in center. Drizzle each steak with sauce and serve with rice.

*See **Specialty Ingredients** (page 34)

NUTRIENT ANALYSIS PER SERVING:

Calories (kcal) 308.81
Protein (g) 41.47
Carbohydrates (g) 11.07
Fat (g) 9.49
Saturated Fat (g) 2.26
Sodium (mg) 500.73

Calories from Protein 173.32
Calories from Carbohydrates 46.25
Calories from Fat 89.24
Cholesterol (mg) 64.60

% Calories from Protein 56.12
% Calories from Carbohydrates 14.98
% Calories from Fat 28.90
Total Dietary Fiber (g) 1.73

GRILLED TUNA WITH MUSTARD SEEDS AND GINGER HONEY MUSTARD SAUCE

∞

This is a fast, flavorful way to serve tuna steaks, and the traditional honey mustard sauce will appeal to everyone.

MAKES 6 SERVINGS

6 six oz. tuna steaks
4 tablespoons yellow or black mustard seeds, ground*
1 tablespoon ground ginger
1 tablespoon brown sugar

SAUCE:

½ cup whole grain mustard
¼ cup honey
2" chunk fresh gingerroot, minced

Fresh jasmine rice for serving (see page 126)

In a shallow pan stir together the ground mustard seeds, ground ginger, and sugar. Coat tuna steaks evenly with spice mixture. Stir together sauce ingredients and set aside. Grill tuna steaks in non-stick grill pan or over coals for 3–5 minutes per side, until just pink in center. Drizzle each steak with sauce and serve with rice.

*Black mustard seeds are available at Indian markets or through the Directory of Resources.

NUTRIENT ANALYSIS PER SERVING:
Calories (kcal) 302.14

Protein (g) 40.17	Calories from Protein 164.30	% Calories from Protein 54.38
Carbohydrates (g) 13.75	Calories from Carbohydrates 56.24	% Calories from Carbohydrates 18.61
Fat (g) 8.87	Calories from Fat 81.60	% Calories from Fat 27.01
Saturated Fat (g) 2.16	Cholesterol (mg) 64.60	Total Dietary Fiber (g) 0.30
Sodium (mg) 67.54		

HONEY GLAZED SESAME TUNA

oney and sesame seeds are a classic Chinese flavor combination, one that suits the rich taste of fresh tuna just perfectly. This dish is terrific with fresh steamed broccoli.

MAKES 2 SERVINGS (EASILY DOUBLED)

2 tablespoons honey

2 tablespoons soy sauce

1½ tablespoons fresh lemon juice

2 teaspoons whole grain dijon mustard

1 tablespoon water

2 teaspoons canola oil

2 six-oz tuna steaks

2 tablespoons toasted sesame seeds*

Jasmine rice for serving (see page 126)

In a small bowl whisk together first five ingredients and set aside. Crush sesame seeds with a mortar and pestle, then spread evenly in a pie plate. Coat the tuna steaks with the crushed seeds. In a large non-stick skillet heat oil over medium high heat, and cook tuna steaks 3–4 minutes per side, until golden and just cooked through. Transfer tuna to serving plates. Add honey glaze to hot skillet and simmer one minute, then pour over tuna. Serve with rice.

*See **Specialty Ingredients** (page 34)

NUTRIENT ANALYSIS PER SERVING:

Calories (kcal) 406.56

Protein (g) 41.95	Calories from Protein 167.87	% Calories from Protein 41.29
Carbohydrates(g) 21.73	Calories from Carbohydrates 86.97	% Calories from Carbohydrates 21.39
Fat (g) 16.85	Calories from Fat 151.72	% Calories from Fat 37.32
Saturated Fat (g) 3.01	Cholesterol (mg) 64.60	Total Dietary Fiber (g) 1.57
Sodium (mg) 601.57		

TANGY LEMON WHITEFISH, CARROTS, AND MUSHROOMS WITH LEMON-SCALLION SAUCE

∞

*T*his recipe evolved from one of my grandmother's traditional one-dish meal recipes. It marries the classic combination of lemon and fish with a delicious vegetable medley. Serve it with plenty of crusty French bread to mop up the extra sauce.

MAKES 4 SERVINGS

> 1 lb. whitefish fillets
> 2 tablespoons canola oil
> 1½ cup diced onion
> 1½ cup diced carrots
> 1½ cup thinly sliced mushrooms
> 2 tablespoons soy cream cheese
> ½ teaspoon dillweed
> ½ teaspoon salt
>
> Fresh crusty French bread for serving

Preheat oven to 350°F. Place fish fillets in 9″ square baking pan. Set aside. In a large saucepan, heat oil over medium heat and add vegetables. Cook, covered, 10 minutes, stirring occasionally, then uncover and cook until liquid evaporates. Stir in all remaining ingredients. Spoon mixture evenly over fish fillets. Cover tightly with foil and bake for 30–35 minutes. Serve with Lemon-Scallion Sauce and crusty French bread.

LEMON-SCALLION SAUCE

¼ cup diced scallions
1 teaspoon canola oil
1½ tablespoon cornstarch
1 cup vegetable broth
Zest from one lemon
Juice from one half lemon

In a small saucepan, sauté scallions in oil until tender. In a small bowl slowly add enough broth to cornstarch to dissolve thoroughly, then stir in remaining broth. Add broth to saucepan and cook over medium high heat until sauce thickens. Add lemon zest and juice and remove from heat.

NUTRIENT ANALYSIS PER SERVING:
Calories (kcal) 282.20

Protein (g) 23.41	Calories from Protein 93.52	% Calories from Protein 33.14
Carbohydrates(g) 12.97	Calories from Carbohydrates 51.80	% Calories from Carbohydrates 18.36
Fat (g) 15.23	Calories from Fat 136.87	% Calories from Fat 48.50
Saturated Fat (g) 1.66	Cholesterol (mg) 68.04	Total Dietary Fiber (g) 2.61
Sodium (mg) 77.44		

SIMPLE WHITEFISH
WITH LEMON AND HERBS
∞

I can't imagine a quicker or easier way to cook fish. This recipe is so simple it's hard to believe the result is practically guaranteed to be delicious. I've tried this with a wide range of fish, and an assortment of dried or fresh herbs (try dill and oregano), and it always turns out fabulous. So go ahead and experiment—this dish is sure to become one of your standbys.

MAKES 4 SERVINGS

> 4 whitefish fillets, about 1½ lbs. total (cod, halibut, etc.)
> 4 large garlic cloves, minced
> 1 teaspoon dried or 4 teaspoons fresh rosemary leaves, crushed
> ¼ teaspoon white pepper
> ¼ teaspoon salt
> 1 tablespoon olive oil
> 1 large lemon, thinly sliced, seeded, end pieces discarded

Preheat oven to 450°F and place a heavy baking sheet in oven to preheat as well. Cut 4 large rectangles of foil or parchment paper* and place a fish fillet in the center of each piece. Combine remaining ingredients except lemon slices in a small bowl and stir well. Spread mixture evenly over fish, scatter lemon slices on top, and fold the edges of the foil or paper up over each fillet, crimping edges tightly.

Place fish packages on preheated baking sheet and bake for 13–15 minutes, until fish is just cooked through. Serve fish in packages.

*Parchment paper is available at some grocery stores and most specialty food stores, health food stores, and kitchen supply shops.

NUTRIENT ANALYSIS PER SERVING:
Calories (kcal) 262.24

Protein (g) 32.66	Calories from Protein 134.44	% Calories from Protein 51.27
Carbohydrates(g) 0.99	Calories from Carbohydrates 4.08	% Calories from Carbohydrates 1.56
Fat (g) 13.36	Calories from Fat 123.71	% Calories from Fat 47.18
Saturated Fat (g) 2.00	Cholesterol (mg) 102.06	Total Dietary Fiber (g) 0.06
Sodium (mg) 232.60		

CHINESE BLACK BEAN STEAMED COD

∞

*I*f you like the black bean sauce served at Chinese restaurants you will love this fish! It's spicy, tangy, and just plain scrumptious.

MAKES 4 SERVINGS

1½ lbs. cod fillets
1 large bunch scallions, cleaned but unchopped

Place fish fillets on top of scallions on a steamer tray, and steam, covered, until fish flakes, about 8 minutes. Transfer to serving platter and discard scallions. Top with spoonfuls of sauce and serve.

SAUCE:

¼ cup black bean garlic sauce (preferably Lee Kum Kee brand)*
¼ cup water
1 tablespoon minced peeled fresh gingerroot
1 teaspoon toasted sesame oil*
2 tablespoons mirin*
2 tablespoons brown sugar

Combine all ingredients in a small bowl and stir well.

*See **Specialty Ingredients** (page 34)

NUTRIENT ANALYSIS PER SERVING:
Calories (kcal) 204.03

Protein (g) 31.01	Calories from Protein 133.72	% Calories from Protein 65.54
Carbohydrates (g) 9.57	Calories from Carbohydrates 41.25	% Calories from Carbohydrates 20.22
Fat (g) 2.99	Calories from Fat 29.06	% Calories from Fat 14.24
Saturated Fat (g) 0.51	Cholesterol (mg) 88.45	Total Dietary Fiber (g) 0.94
Sodium (mg) 129.19		

CHABLIS CHICKEN
∞

another traditional recipe from my grandmother, this chicken didn't need a single modification for the IBS kitchen. It's perfectly safe and utterly delicious just the way it is.

MAKES 6 SERVINGS

3 whole organic chicken breasts, skinless and boneless
½ teaspoon salt
¼ teaspoon freshly ground black pepper
2 tablespoons canola oil
1 cup Chablis wine
½ cup apple jelly
½ cup currants, diced

Cooked rice for serving

Sprinkle chicken with salt and pepper and set aside. In a large non-stick skillet heat oil over medium heat and cook chicken until golden brown, about four minutes per side. Remove chicken from skillet. Add to skillet Chablis, apple jelly, and currants, and simmer, stirring constantly, until bubbly and smooth. Return chicken to skillet and baste with sauce. Cover pan and simmer 20–30 minutes or until chicken is just cooked through. Serve with rice.

NUTRIENT ANALYSIS PER SERVING:
Calories (kcal) 267.97

Protein (g) 12.89	Calories from Protein 58.37	% Calories from Protein 21.78
Carbohydrates (g) 28.74	Calories from Carbohydrates 130.15	% Calories from Carbohydrates 48.57
Fat (g) 7.80	Calories from Fat 79.45	% Calories from Fat 29.65
Saturated Fat (g) 0.68	Cholesterol (mg) 30.89	Total Dietary Fiber (g)* 0.44
Sodium (mg) 344.53		

LACQUERED FIVE-SPICE CHICKEN
∞

*T*his is an adaptation of a recipe my grandmother learned at an Asian cooking class back when I was a little girl. It was a family favorite for many years. The chicken is tender and spicy but not hot, and the marinade has an exotic complexity of flavors that belie the simple preparation. Serve with plenty of rose rice to soak up the extra sauce.

MAKES 4 SERVINGS

> 4 organic skinless, boneless chicken breasts
> 1 three inch piece fresh gingerroot, skinned
> ¼ cup shoyu* (a type of soy sauce)
> 2 tablespoons water
> ¼ teaspoon five-spice powder*
> 1 tablespoon canola oil
> 2 cloves minced garlic
> 1 teaspoon honey
> Several whole star anise*
>
> Freshly shredded lettuce leaves to serve
>
> Cooked rose rice to serve (see page 125)

Preheat oven to 350°F. Rub the chicken thoroughly with the ginger. Mince the ginger and add it to the remaining ingredients to make a marinade. Add chicken to marinade and chill, 1 hour, turning over once. Add chicken with marinade to 9″ square baking pan, and bake, covered, for 45–55 minutes, basting frequently, until chicken is just cooked through. Turn chicken once or twice. Add water as needed to sauce if it becomes too thick. Serve chicken over shredded lettuce, with rose rice and additional sauce.

*Shoyu, five-spice powder, and whole star anise are available in the Asian section of many grocery stores, at Asian markets, at some health food stores, or see Directory of Resources.

NUTRIENT ANALYSIS PER SERVING:
Calories (kcal) 294.17

Protein (g) 53.20	Calories from Protein 222.86	% Calories from Protein 75.76
Carbohydrates (g) 2.80	Calories from Carbohydrates 11.71	% Calories from Carbohydrates 3.98
Fat (g) 6.32	Calories from Fat 59.60	% Calories from Fat 20.26
Saturated Fat (g) 1.00	Cholesterol (mg) 131.54	Total Dietary Fiber (g) 0.13
Sodium (mg) 677.44		

SIMPLE HERB BAKED
CHICKEN BREASTS

∞

*W*hen you feel like an old-fashioned Thanksgiving dinner but aren't up to roasting a turkey, try this recipe with Maple-Glazed Red Cabbage (page 124) and Old-Fashioned Bread Stuffing with Dried Apricots and Currants (page 135). For an over-the-top finale bake some Pumpkin Spice Pie with Praline Topping (page 252) for dessert.

MAKES 4 SERVINGS

4 organic skinless chicken breasts with bone
4 teaspoons olive oil

HERB RUB:

1 teaspoon dried crushed thyme
1 crushed bay leaf
1 teaspoon dried crushed basil
1 teaspoon rubbed sage
¼ teaspoon white pepper

Preheat oven to 300°F. Place the chicken on a broiling rack in a large shallow pan. Brush each breast with 1 teaspoon olive oil and rub generously with herb mix. Bake 40 minutes, covered with foil, basting occasionally.

NUTRIENT ANALYSIS PER SERVING:
Calories (kcal) 117.88

Protein (g) 16.39	Calories from Protein 67.81	% Calories from Protein 57.52
Fat (g) 5.38	Calories from Fat 50.07	% Calories from Fat 42.48
Saturated Fat (g) 0.84	Cholesterol (mg) 41.18	Sodium (mg) 46.15

EASY PEACHY CHICKEN BREASTS

∞

*T*he chipotle peppers in this dish don't add heat but they do add a wonderful smoky nuance to the sweetness of the peaches. The combination is outstanding.

MAKES 4 SERVINGS

2 whole organic chicken breasts, boneless and skinless
1 tablespoon olive oil
3 firm-ripe fresh peaches, pitted and quartered
3 medium onions, chopped
½ teaspoon ground chipotle pepper,* or to taste
6 large garlic cloves
1 lemon, quartered

Brown rice for serving

Preheat oven to 375°F. Place chicken breasts in an 18 x 11½" roasting pan, and season with salt and pepper. Drizzle with oil, scatter remaining ingredients evenly over chicken, cover with foil, and roast at 375°F for 20 minutes. Remove foil and roast chicken, basting occasionally, for 20 minutes, or until cooked through. Serve chicken over rice, spooning pan juices on top.

*See **Specialty Ingredients** (page 34)

NUTRIENT ANALYSIS PER SERVING:
Calories (kcal) 118.75

Protein (g) 9.32	Calories from Protein 36.28	% Calories from Protein 30.55
Carbohydrates (g) 12.02	Calories from Carbohydrates 46.80	% Calories from Carbohydrates 39.41
Fat (g) 4.07	Calories from Fat 35.68	% Calories from Fat 30.04
Saturated Fat (g) 0.38	Cholesterol (mg) 20.59	Total Dietary Fiber (g) 2.06
Sodium (mg) 24.67		

THAI-GRILLED CHICKEN SATAYS
WITH SWEET AND TANGY
DIPPING SAUCE
∞

his is one of my most-requested recipes. Thai satays are traditionally served with a peanut-coconut milk sauce—delicious, but deadly. This sweet chili sauce is a much safer, and equally scrumptious, alternative. Try some Spring Blossom Tea (page 44) as the perfect Thai accompaniment.

MAKES 6 SERVINGS

2 lbs. organic skinless, boneless chicken breasts

In a glass pie plate make a marinade of:
2 tablespoons brown sugar
2 tablespoons Thai or Vietnamese fish sauce*
1 tablespoon ground coriander seeds
1″ chunk fresh gingerroot, minced
1 small stalk fresh lemongrass, lower stalk trimmed to 3 inches and very finely sliced*
2 teaspoons curry powder
¼ teaspoon cumin
3 tablespoons fresh lemon juice
2 tablespoons soy sauce
2 tablespoons canola oil
4 cloves garlic, minced

Cooked rose rice for serving (see page 125)
Asian Sweet Pickled Cucumbers for serving (see page 123)
Sweet and Tangy Dipping Sauce for serving (see page 176)

Slice chicken breasts in half horizontally, then cut into long strips 1″ wide. Add to marinade, cover, and chill for at least 4 hours and up to 24 hours. Place chicken strips on broiler pan, and broil under high heat, turning once or twice, until just cooked through, about 3–4 minutes total. Alternately, chicken can be grilled instead of broiled.

Serve immediately over rose rice with Sweet and Tangy Dipping Sauce and Asian Sweet Pickled Cucumbers.

*See **Specialty Ingredients** (page 34)

NUTRIENT ANALYSIS PER SERVING:
Calories (kcal) 297.07

Protein (g) 35.68	Calories from Protein 144.36	% Calories from Protein 48.60
Carbohydrates (g) 22.99	Calories from Carbohydrates 93.02	% Calories from Carbohydrates 31.31
Fat (g) 6.56	Calories from Fat 59.69	% Calories from Fat 20.09
Saturated Fat (g) 0.83	Cholesterol (mg) 87.70	Total Dietary Fiber (g) 0.12
Sodium (mg) 860.39		

CHARGRILLED VIETNAMESE CHICKEN WITH RICE NOODLES AND LIME DIPPING SAUCE

∞

*R*ice noodles marry perfectly with Vietnamese marinades—their bland chewiness is the perfect foil for those tart and tangy lime sauces. The addition of smoky grilled chicken and the bright flavors of fresh mint and basil finish this dish deliciously.

MAKES 6 SERVINGS

4 organic skinless, boneless chicken breasts (about 1 lb. total)
3 tablespoons packed brown sugar
2 tablespoons soy sauce
1 teaspoon garlic powder
1 lb. rice-stick noodles*
2 carrots, finely shredded
½ cup fresh mint leaves, finely chopped
¼ cup finely chopped scallions
¼ cup honey

Cut chicken into one-inch pieces and thread onto metal skewers without crowding. In a shallow pie plate large enough to hold skewers in one layer, whisk together brown sugar, soy sauce, and garlic powder. Add chicken, turn to coat, and marinate for 30 minutes, turning occasionally.

Fill a large kettle with water and bring to boil. Add noodles and cook, stirring occasionally, for 5 minutes, or until tender. Drain noodles and rinse under cold water. Transfer noodles to serving platter, and toss with carrot, mint, and scallions.

Remove chicken skewers from marinade, brush with honey, and grill over coals or in grill pan, turning frequently, until chicken is cooked through, about 10 minutes. Remove chicken from skewers and place on top of rice noodle mixture. Drizzle with dipping sauce and pass additional sauce at the table.

LIME DIPPING SAUCE:

⅓ cup Thai or Vietnamese fish sauce**
½ cup fresh lime juice
½ cup granulated sugar
1 cup boiling water

In a small bowl whisk together all ingredients.

*Available at Asian markets, or see Directory of Resources

See **Specialty Ingredients (page 34)

NUTRIENT ANALYSIS PER SERVING:
Calories (kcal) 485.27

Protein (g) 15.03	Calories from Protein 60.39	% Calories from Protein 12.44
Carbohydrates (g) 103.31	Calories from Carbohydrates 415.09	% Calories from Carbohydrates 85.54
Fat (g) 1.08	Calories from Fat 9.79	% Calories from Fat 2.02
Saturated Fat (g) 0.28	Cholesterol (mg) 27.45	Total Dietary Fiber (g) 2.09
Sodium (mg) 1615.57		

JAMAICAN CHICKEN WITH GINGER PEACH CHUTNEY

∞

bsolutely perfect for a backyard barbecue or beach picnic! Serve this chicken hot or cold, with jasmine rice and Virgin Strawberry Daiquiris (page 52). Your guests will thank you, your family will love you, and everyone will enjoy a little taste of the tropics. For a fun change of pace I make this dish in the dead of winter, crank up the heat, put on some shorts, and play reggae music. It's cheaper than flying to the Caribbean and just as tasty.

MAKES 6 SERVINGS (DOUBLES OR TRIPLES EASILY)

4 organic boneless skinless chicken breasts, rinsed and patted dry
Cooked jasmine rice for serving

In a medium bowl, stir together seasoning mix:
 1 teaspoon chili powder
 1 teaspoon garlic powder
 1 teaspoon dried basil
 1 teaspoon dried thyme
 1 teaspoon ground coriander
 1 teaspoon ground ginger
 1 teaspoon allspice
 ½ teaspoon cinnamon
 ½ teaspoon ground cloves
 ½ teaspoon black pepper
 ½ teaspoon nutmeg
 1 tablespoon granulated sugar

Add to seasoning mix:
 ½ cup fresh orange juice
 2 tablespoons olive oil
 Juice of 1 lime
 1 cup finely diced onion

Stir well to make a marinade. Transfer marinade to a glass pie plate, add chicken breasts, cover, and marinate overnight. Grill for 5–6 minutes per side, just until done, basting with marinade.

Serve with jasmine rice and Ginger Peach Chutney.

GINGER PEACH CHUTNEY:

4 large ripe peaches, peeled, pitted, and diced
⅔ cup fresh pineapple, diced
2 inch chunk of fresh gingerroot, peeled and minced
½ cup diced onion
½ teaspoon ground coriander
¼ teaspoon ground cumin
2 tablespoons honey
½ cup fresh orange juice
Salt and pepper to taste

Combine all ingredients in a large heavy saucepan and simmer, uncovered, until peaches cook down and liquid evaporates, about 30–40 minutes. Chill for at least one day to marry flavors. Chutney freezes well in an airtight container.

NUTRIENT ANALYSIS PER SERVING:
Calories (kcal) 191.17

Protein (g) 12.19	Calories from Protein 47.23	% Calories from Protein 24.71
Carbohydrates(g) 25.09	Calories from Carbohydrates 97.19	% Calories from Carbohydrates 50.84
Fat (g) 5.36	Calories from Fat 46.75	% Calories from Fat 24.45
Saturated Fat (g) 0.79	Cholesterol (mg) 27.45	Total Dietary Fiber (g) 2.26
Sodium (mg) 32.76		

VIETNAMESE LEMONGRASS GINGER CHICKEN

∞

*T*his is a classic Vietnamese restaurant recipe and my husband's favorite. It's fast, easy, and the lemongrass gives it an interesting twist.

MAKES 4 SERVINGS

2 organic boneless, skinless chicken breasts
2 tablespoons canola oil
6 cloves minced garlic
2 large onions, diced
1 large carrot, diced
1 teaspoon salt
1 teaspoon chili powder
1 inch piece of fresh gingerroot, minced
3 large stalks fresh lemongrass, bottom 3 inches of stalks trimmed and finely minced*
1 tablespoon Thai or Vietnamese fish sauce*
1 tablespoon brown sugar
¼ cup Caramel Sauce
1 cup water
2 scallions, diced

Fresh cilantro leaves for serving
Cooked jasmine rice for serving (see page 126)

Rinse chicken, pat dry, and cut into bite size pieces. Set aside. Heat oil in a large non-stick skillet over medium heat, add garlic, onions, and carrots, and sauté until soft. Add salt, chili powder, ginger, and lemongrass. Sauté until fragrant, about 2 minutes. Add chicken and cook until slightly browned. Add fish sauce, sugar, and Caramel Sauce. Stir well. Add water and scallions and cook, covered, just until chicken is tender. Top with fresh cilantro leaves and serve with jasmine rice.

CARAMEL SAUCE:

½ cup granulated sugar
4 tablespoons water

Mix sugar and water in a small heavy saucepan. Bring to a boil and cook until mixture changes color. Reduce heat to low and cook until brown. Add an additional ½ cup water and remove from heat. Sauce keeps indefinitely in refrigerator.

*See **Specialty Ingredients** (page 34)

NUTRIENT ANALYSIS PER SERVING:
Calories (kcal) 211.90

Protein (g) 10.89	Calories from Protein 42.69	% Calories from Protein 20.15
Carbohydrates (g) 25.99	Calories from Carbohydrates 101.87	% Calories from Carbohydrates 48.08
Fat (g) 7.63	Calories from Fat 67.33	% Calories from Fat 31.78
Saturated Fat (g) 0.65	Cholesterol (mg) 20.59	Total Dietary Fiber (g) 2.18
Sodium (mg) 2468.76		

ORANGE-GLAZED CHICKEN BREASTS WITH ONIONS, MUSHROOMS, AND CARROTS

∞

*H*ere's a traditional homestyle chicken dinner that will be loved by everyone.

MAKES 4 SERVINGS

> 2 tablespoons cornstarch
> ½ teaspoon white pepper
> 1 tablespoon paprika
> 3 whole organic chicken breasts, skinless and boneless, chopped into bite-size pieces
> 2 tablespoons canola oil
> 1 cup chopped onion
> ½ cup chopped carrots
> ½ cup sautéed and drained mushrooms
> 1 tablespoon brown sugar
> ¼ teaspoon ginger
> ⅓ cup undiluted frozen orange juice concentrate, thawed
> ¾ cup water
>
> Jasmine rice for serving (see page 126)

Preheat oven to 350°F. Combine cornstarch, pepper, and paprika in a plastic bag. Add chicken pieces and shake until well-coated. Reserve coating mixture. Heat oil in a large non-stick skillet over medium high heat and cook chicken until browned on all sides. Remove chicken from skillet and add to a 2 quart casserole dish. Add onions, carrots, and mushrooms to casserole dish.

Blend reserved coating mix and remaining ingredients into skillet with drippings. Cook over medium heat, stirring constantly, until smooth and bubbly. Pour sauce over chicken, cover, and bake for 45–55 minutes, until chicken is just cooked through. Serve with rice.

NUTRIENT ANALYSIS PER SERVING:
Calories (kcal) 213.82

Protein (g) 14.17	Calories from Protein 55.83	% Calories from Protein 26.11
Carbohydrates (g) 21.84	Calories from Carbohydrates 86.03	% Calories from Carbohydrates 40.23
Fat (g) 8.12	Calories from Fat 71.96	% Calories from Fat 33.66
Saturated Fat (g) 0.74	Cholesterol (mg) 30.89	Total Dietary Fiber (g) 2.20
Sodium (mg) 44.07		

BENGALI SPICED CHICKPEAS, TOMATOES, AND SPINACH WITH BLACK SALT

∞

*T*his vegetarian dish is hearty, tasty, nutritious, and packed with soluble fiber. The black salt is worth hunting for as it adds a unique tang that makes this recipe memorable. Serve this with Indian Pistachio Orange Blossom Tapioca Pudding (page 232) for dessert and you will have yourself an ethnic feast.

MAKES 4 SERVINGS

I tablespoon olive oil
I teaspoon black mustard seeds*
½ teaspoon asafoetida powder*
I tablespoon mild curry powder
¼ teaspoon ground cumin
¼ teaspoon ground coriander
I cup chopped onion
4 large garlic cloves, minced
10 oz. spinach (about one small bunch), cooked, drained, and chopped fine
8 oz. can tomato sauce
19 oz. cooked or canned chickpeas, rinsed and drained, divided
I cup vegetable stock
Black salt to taste*

Basmati rice for serving (see page 126)

In a large skillet heat the oil over medium high, add the spices, and cook, stirring until the mustard seeds pop and the spices are fragrant. Add the onion and garlic and sauté until golden, about five minutes. Add the spinach, tomato sauce, and 1 cup chickpeas. In a blender, purée the remaining chickpeas with the broth. Add the puréed chickpeas to the skillet and simmer, stirring occasionally, until hot. Add black salt to taste and serve with rice.

*Available at Indian markets or see Directory of Resources

NUTRIENT ANALYSIS PER SERVING:
Calories (kcal) 303.80

Protein (g) 15.44	Calories from Protein 58.52	% Calories from Protein 19.26
Carbohydrates (g) 47.85	Calories from Carbohydrates 181.42	% Calories from Carbohydrates 59.72
Fat (g) 7.49	Calories from Fat 63.86	% Calories from Fat 21.02
Saturated Fat (g) 0.92	Total Dietary Fiber (g) 14.05	Sodium (mg) 410.65

FAT RICE NOODLES WITH SWEET BLACK SOY SAUCE, SCALLIONS, AND PRAWNS

∞

his is a wonderful Thai dish that is worth a trip to an Asian market for the special ingredi-ents. The sweet black soy sauce carmelizes in the wok to create a rich smoky sweetness that coats the noodles delectably. The prawns and scallions add pretty notes of color and contrast, and make this a favorite one-dish meal.

MAKES 4-5 SERVINGS

Two 12 oz. packages presliced fresh rice noodles*
2 tablespoons canola oil
1 whole head of garlic cloves, mashed
6 tablespoons water, or as needed
3 tablespoons sweet black soy sauce*
6 tablespoons mushroom soy sauce (Healthy Boy brand)*
½ cup plus 1 tablespoon brown sugar
¼–½ teaspoon white pepper, or to taste
1 lb. prawns, shelled and deveined
1 medium bunch scallions, trimmed and diced

Place the rice noodles in a colander and pour hot water over them to separate and slightly soften. Separate noodles as much as possible.

Set a wok over medium high heat and add oil. When oil is hot add the garlic and stir fry until golden. Add the water and noodles and stir fry one minute. Add the sweet black soy sauce and stir until well blended. Add the mushroom soy sauce, sugar, and white pepper and stir fry until the sugar is dissolved. Add the prawns and scallions and stir fry until the prawns are pink and just cooked through and the scallions are tender. Serve immediately

*See **Kitchen Essentials** (page 31)

NUTRIENT ANALYSIS PER SERVING:
Calories (kcal) 399.36

Protein (g) 21.06	Calories from Protein 85.27	% Calories from Protein 21.35
Carbohydrates (g) 60.71	Calories from Carbohydrates 245.86	% Calories from Carbohydrates 61.56
Fat (g) 7.49	Calories from Fat 68.22	% Calories from Fat 17.08
Saturated Fat (g) 0.73	Cholesterol (mg) 137.89	Total Dietary Fiber (g) 1.92
Sodium (mg) 895.37		

INDIAN CURRIED POTATOES, PEAS, AND CARROTS

∞

I absolutely love this recipe, and make it quite often for a vegetarian dinner. It is very flavorful and spicy but not at all hot, and the leftovers make a workday lunch to die for. This dish is perfect with Sweet Cardamom and Currant Indian Rice (page 128), pappadams, and mango chutney.

MAKES 4 SERVINGS

> 2 tablespoons canola oil, divided
> 1 tablespoon whole cumin seeds
> 1 tablespoon black mustard seeds*
> 1 tablespoon asofoetida powder*
> 2 cups thinly sliced onions
> 1 teaspoon ground turmeric
> 1 teaspoon chili powder
> 1 teaspoon ground coriander
> 1 teaspoon salt
> 1½ lbs. new potatoes, peeled and cut into ¼" slices
> ½ lb. carrots (about 4), cut into ¼" slices
> 1–2 cups water, as needed
> 1 cup fresh or frozen peas
>
> Fresh cilantro for garnish

In a large heavy skillet heat 1 tablespoon of oil over high heat add the cumin and mustard seeds. Cook 30–60 seconds, until they pop and blacken. Reduce heat to medium, stir in the asofoetida powder, and add the remaining 1 tablespoon of oil. Add the onions and cook until golden, about 10–15 minutes.

Stir in the turmeric, chili powder, coriander and salt. Reduce heat to low and add the potatoes and carrots. Add enough water to cover bottom of skillet, cover, and cook until vegetables are tender. Stir occasionally and add additional water as needed to keep mixture from burning. Add peas, cover, and cook until peas are tender, about 5 minutes. Serve garnished with fresh cilantro.

*Available at Indian markets or through the Directory of Resources

Nutrient Analysis Per Serving:
Calories (kcal) 276.09

Protein (g) 6.92	Calories from Protein 26.80	% Calories from Protein 9.71
Carbohydrates(g) 47.55	Calories from Carbohydrates 184.27	% Calories from Carbohydrates 66.74
Fat (g) 7.46	Calories from Fat 65.02	% Calories from Fat 23.55
Saturated Fat (g) 0.59	Total Dietary Fiber (g) 7.66	Sodium (mg) 614.35

GARDEN VEGGIE LO MEIN

This Cantonese-style lo mein has a wonderful smoky flavor that comes from a smidgen of sesame oil. Because sesame oil has a low smoking point, it is usually unsuitable for stirfries, but in this recipe it is used for that very reason. Just a tiny bit provides great flavor, and a dash of soy sauce finishes this dish nicely. Lo mein makes a wonderfully nutritious vegetarian dinner that comes together quite quickly on those weekday evenings when you don't have much time or energy to cook. This recipe was inspired by the delicious lomein that is a specialty of Sifu Winchell Woo, a Kung Fu teacher and extraordinary chef—and a very nice guy, too.

MAKES 6 SERVINGS

1 lb. package of fresh Chinese lo mein noodles*
2 teaspoons canola oil
1 teaspoon sesame oil
1 large garlic clove, minced
1" chunk fresh gingerroot, peeled and minced
1 medium onion, roughly chopped
1 cup coarsely shredded carrots
1½ cups coarsely shredded peeled zucchini
4 scallions, trimmed and sliced into one-inch lengths
Soy sauce to taste (try Jen Mai)
White pepper to taste

Bring a large pot of water to boil and add the lo mein noodles, cooking until slightly tender but still quite chewy, about 1–2 minutes. Drain and rinse, then spray noodles with cooking oil. Run your fingers through the noodles to separate the strands and distribute the oil, spraying a little more oil throughout the noodles to evenly coat them. Cut the noodles into shorter lengths with kitchen shears.

Heat the canola and sesame oil in a wok over high heat until it just smokes. Add the garlic and ginger and stir fry just until fragrant, about 1 minute. Add the noodles and stir fry until golden. Remove noodles from wok and set aside. Add the vegetables and stir fry until crisp-tender. Add the noodles back to the wok and cook until they are just tender and have absorbed the liquid from the vegetables. Stir in soy sauce and white pepper to taste and serve.

*Available at Asian markets or see Directory of Resources

NUTRIENT ANALYSIS PER SERVING:

Calories (kcal) 482.14

Protein (g) 15.75	Calories from Protein 63.46	% Calories from Protein 13.16
Carbohydrates (g) 91.67	Calories from Carbohydrates 369.42	% Calories from Carbohydrates 76.62
Fat (g) 5.43	Calories from Fat 49.26	% Calories from Fat 10.22
Saturated Fat (g) 0.61	Total Dietary Fiber (g) 4.76	Sodium (mg) 20.78

JAPANESE SOBA NOODLES WITH BONITO DIPPING SAUCE AND TOASTED NORI

∞

*I*f you've never had soba noodles before, this dinner will be a real treat. They have a very hearty flavor that comes from buckwheat flour, and they're traditionally served chilled. Soba noodles are a staple in my house for fast, easy dinners; they're delicious served with steamed sweet potatoes or fresh soybeans.

MAKES 4 SERVINGS

DIPPING SAUCE:

⅓ cup boiling water
¼ cup bonito flakes*
2 tablespoons Japanese soy sauce, such as Kikkoman's
2 tablespoons granulated sugar

6 oz. dried soba noodles*
1 sheet nori seaweed,* cut into thin strips with kitchen shears
Toasted sesame seeds**

Combine boiling water and bonito flakes, and set aside for 10 minutes. Strain broth, pressing hard on solids, and discard bonito. Stir soy sauce and sugar into broth until dissolved. Set aside.

Bring a large pot of water to boil and add the noodles, cooking, stirring occasionally, until tender, about 10 minutes. Drain and rinse with cold water until chilled. Divide noodles among serving bowls and sprinkle with shredded nori and toasted sesame seeds. Serve with dipping sauce.

*Available at Asian markets or see Directory of Resources

See **Specialty Ingredients (page 34)

NUTRIENT ANALYSIS PER SERVING:
Calories (kcal) 184.13

Protein (g) 6.95	Calories from Protein 25.97	% Calories from Protein 14.10
Carbohydrates (g) 39.48	Calories from Carbohydrates 147.48	% Calories from Carbohydrates 80.09
Fat (g) 1.27	Calories from Fat 10.68	% Calories from Fat 5.80
Saturated Fat (g) 0.19	Total Dietary Fiber (g) 0.41	Sodium (mg) 639.39

LINGUINE WITH CALAMARI
AND GARLIC WHITE WINE SAUCE

Here's a traditional Italian pasta meal that's both scrumptious and safe.

MAKES 6-8 SERVINGS

16 oz. dried linguine
1 tablespoon olive oil
8 anchovies, rinsed of oil and drained
6 large garlic cloves, minced
¼ cup capers
1½ cups dry white wine
½ cup packed basil leaves, finely shredded
1 lb. squid steaks, cut into rings

Cook pasta in a large pot of boiling water until just tender but still firm to bite. Drain pasta, reserving 1 cup cooking water.

In a large non-stick skillet heat the olive oil and sauté anchovies and garlic until anchovies melt and garlic is golden. Stir in the capers and wine and boil until sauce is slightly reduced, about 3 minutes. Stir in basil. Reduce heat to medium low and add calamari, cooking and stirring until just opaque. Do not overcook or calamari will be tough. Add pasta to skillet, tossing until heated through adding reserved pasta cooking water as necessary. Serve immediately.

NUTRIENT ANALYSIS PER SERVING:
Calories (kcal) 427.03

Protein (g) 23.37	Calories from Protein 104.69	% Calories from Protein 24.52
Carbohydrates (g) 60.54	Calories from Carbohydrates 271.22	% Calories from Carbohydrates 63.51
Fat (g) 5.07	Calories from Fat 51.11	% Calories from Fat 11.97
Saturated Fat (g) 0.88	Cholesterol (mg) 180.68	Total Dietary Fiber (g) 2.06
Sodium (mg) 407.58		

FETTUCINE WITH CREAMY
BUTTERNUT SQUASH SAUCE

*his is an unusual vegetarian fettucine, with a slightly sweet and nutty sauce. It's just as nutri-
tious as it is delicious, so give it a try when you're in the mood for something a little different.*

MAKES 6-8 SERVINGS

> 4 cups fresh or frozen butternut squash, peeled, diced, and steamed until very
>   tender
> 2 cups plain soy milk
> 2 tablespoons cornstarch
> 2 tablespoons olive oil
> 2 cups diced onion
> 4 garlic cloves, minced
> 1 teaspoon dried rosemary
> 2 teaspoons dried savory
> 2 teaspoons dried basil
> 1 teaspoon salt
> 2 teaspoons brown sugar
> 16 oz. package linguine, cooked, 1 cup cooking water reserved
> Soy Parmesan

Whisk together the steamed squash, soy milk, and cornstarch until smooth. Set aside.
Heat olive oil in a large nonstick skillet. Sauté onion, garlic, and herbs until very tender
and golden. Add the squash mixture, salt, and sugar, and cook over medium low heat
until the sauce thickens. If sauce is too heavy add some reserved pasta water. Spoon the
sauce over the cooked linguine and top with soy Parmesan.

NUTRIENT ANALYSIS PER SERVING:
Calories (kcal) 440.52

Protein (g) 13.94	Calories from Protein 54.83	% Calories from Protein 12.45
Carbohydrates (g) 81.25	Calories from Carbohydrates 319.51	% Calories from Carbohydrates 72.53
Fat (g) 7.48	Calories from Fat 66.19	% Calories from Fat 15.03
Saturated Fat (g) 1.00	Total Dietary Fiber (g)* 3.91	Sodium (mg) 733.27

SPAGHETTI WITH SPANISH ALMOND ROMESCO SAUCE

∞

*T*his recipe is a wonderful way to use a bounty of summertime ripe tomatoes. It's a delicious change of pace from traditional spaghetti sauce.

MAKES 6-8 SERVINGS

2 large, thick slices French bread, cut into ½" cubes
¼ cup white vinegar
¼ cup Balsamic vinegar
¾ cup sliced almonds
1 lb. whole ripe tomatoes, roasted or broiled until skins blacken (about 4–6 tomatoes)
1 tablespoon paprika
1 large garlic clove, minced
¼ teaspoon salt
¼ teaspoon ground black pepper
3 tablespoons extra-virgin olive oil

1 lb. cooked spaghetti for serving

In a medium bowl, soak the bread in the vinegars for 20 minutes. In a large, dry hot non-stick skillet toast the almonds until golden brown, stirring frequently and watching closely. Cool the almonds and grind in a food processor until they are fine crumbs, but not oily. Add the soaked bread, tomatoes, paprika, garlic, salt, and pepper to the processor and mix briefly until evenly puréed. Add the olive oil in a thin stream until just incorporated.

Serve sauce with hot spaghetti.

Leftover sauce will keep, refrigerated, for one week. It can also be frozen for several months.

NUTRIENT ANALYSIS PER SERVING:
Calories (kcal) 496.82

Protein (g) 15.03	Calories from Protein 59.16	% Calories from Protein 11.91
Carbohydrates(g) 70.53	Calories from Carbohydrates 277.63	% Calories from Carbohydrates 55.88
Fat (g) 18.07	Calories from Fat 160.02	% Calories from Fat 32.21
Saturated Fat (g) 2.09	Total Dietary Fiber (g) 4.21	Sodium (mg) 181.51

LINGUINE WITH CREAMY WILD MUSHROOM, SPINACH, AND SHERRY SAUCE

∞

This pasta is elegantly rich and hearty. If you thought you could never enjoy a luscious cream sauce again this recipe will prove you deliciously wrong.

MAKES 4-6 SERVINGS

12 oz. dried linguine
2 tablespoons olive oil
1 medium onions, diced
4 cups mixed wild mushrooms, thinly sliced
3 tablespoons whole wheat pastry flour
1⅓ cups plain rice milk
1 teaspoon whole grain Dijon mustard
1 teaspoon marjoram
1 cup packed shredded spinach leaves
½ cup Sherry or white wine
Salt and pepper to taste

Fresh crusty French bread for serving

Cook the linguine in boiling water until tender, reserve ½ cup cooking water, drain linguine, and set aside.

Heat olive oil in a large non-stick frying pan and sauté the onion until softened. Add the mushrooms and cook until the liquid they release has mostly evaporated and the mushrooms are tender. Sift the flour into the pan and stir thoroughly. Slowly add the rice milk, stirring constantly, and heat until the sauce just boils and has thickened. Lower heat, add remaining ingredients, and simmer until spinach is thoroughly cooked and incorporated into sauce. Add the cooked pasta to the pan, stir well to combine, adding reserved pasta cooking water if necessary, and serve immediately with French bread.

NUTRIENT ANALYSIS PER SERVING:
Calories (kcal) 489.64

Protein (g) 16.28	Calories from Protein 70.27	% Calories from Protein 14.35
Carbohydrates(g) 73.23	Calories from Carbohydrates 316.09	% Calories from Carbohydrates 64.56
Fat (g) 10.63	Calories from Fat 103.28	% Calories from Fat 21.09
Saturated Fat (g) 1.40	Total Dietary Fiber (g)* 5.92	Sodium (mg) 39.24

CRISPY PIZZA
WITH SEAFOOD AND DILL
∞

*O*h, *who doesn't love pizza? I sure do, but the traditional version that's loaded with meat and cheese just kills me. Is there such a thing as good pizza without pepperoni and mozzarella? Of course there is! You can top a pizza with just about anything, as long as it's low fat, because the crust provides a good soluble fiber base. Try a wide range of cooked vegetables, chicken, or seafood, and be creative with your sauces. This version, with shrimp, crab, and dill, is as delicious as it is safe.*

MAKES TWO 16" PIZZAS, 8 SLICES PER PIZZA

PIZZA DOUGH:

1½ cup warm water (105–115°F)
1 tablespoon active dry yeast
4 cups all-purpose unbleached white flour
2 teaspoons salt

In a small bowl stir together water and yeast until yeast dissolves. In a large bowl whisk together flour and salt and add yeast liquid, stirring with a wooden spoon until a soft dough forms. Knead dough until smooth and elastic, about 10 minutes, on a lightly floured surface.

Spray a large bowl lightly with cooking oil and transfer dough to bowl. Cover with plastic wrap and a kitchen towel, and let dough rise in a warm, (about 75-85°) draft-free place until doubled in bulk, about 1½ hours.

Punch down dough and cut into two pieces, then form each piece into a ball. Put each ball of dough into a separate, lightly oiled large bowl and cover each bowl with a kitchen towel. Place bowls in a warm (about 75–85°) draft-free place, and let dough rise until again doubled in bulk, about 1 hour.

Roll out each ball of dough separately into a 16″ circle and transfer dough to pizza pans or stones.

TOPPING:

Olive oil
¾ cup shelled and deveined raw prawns
¾ cup crab meat or surimi*
1 tablespoon dill
2 tablespoons chopped capers

Preheat oven to 450°F. Brush dough very lightly with olive oil. Bake untopped dough for 5–7 minutes or until it is dry but not browning. Remove from oven, sprinkle evenly with toppings, and bake for another 5–7 minutes or until crisp at center and prawns are cooked through.

*See **Specialty Ingredients** (page 34)

NUTRIENT ANALYSIS PER SLICE:
Calories (kcal) 130.59

Protein (g) 6.32	Calories from Protein 25.84	% Calories from Protein 19.79
Carbohydrates (g) 24.29	Calories from Carbohydrates 99.29	% Calories from Carbohydrates 76.03
Fat (g) 0.59	Calories from Fat 5.46	% Calories from Fat 4.18
Saturated Fat (g) 0.10	Cholesterol (mg) 17.88	Total Dietary Fiber (g) 1.05
Sodium (mg) 366.94		

Pizza with Fresh Basil, Grilled Chicken, Roasted Garlic, and Sundried Tomatoes

∞

*H*ere's a wonderful summertime pizza that smells just incredible as it bakes.

MAKES TWO 16" PIZZAS, 8 SLICES PER PIZZA

Follow pizza dough instructions on page 219.

TOPPING:

I head of garlic, wrapped in foil and roasted at 400°F for 45 minutes, or until
   soft
⅔ cup sun-dried tomatoes, soaked in boiling hot water for 15 minutes then
   drained
I cup grilled shredded skinless organic chicken breasts
⅓ cup packed fresh basil leaves, finely shredded

Preheat oven to 450°F. Brush dough very lightly with olive oil. Squeeze garlic cloves
from skins and mix in a small bowl with drained sun-dried tomatoes. Bake untopped
dough for 5–7 minutes or until it is dry but not browning. Remove from oven, sprinkle evenly with roasted garlic, tomatoes, and chicken, and bake for another 5–7 minutes. Remove from oven and top with shredded basil.

NUTRIENT ANALYSIS PER SLICE:
Calories (kcal) 130.17

Protein (g) 4.90	Calories from Protein 19.78	% Calories from Protein 15.20
Carbohydrates (g) 26.17	Calories from Carbohydrates 105.59	% Calories from Carbohydrates 81.12
Fat (g) 0.53	Calories from Fat 4.80	% Calories from Fat 3.68
Saturated Fat (g) 0.09	Cholesterol (mg) 2.48	Total Dietary Fiber (g) 1.36
Sodium (mg) 341.40		

CRISPY PIZZA WITH SHREDDED CHICKEN, SCALLIONS, AND SMOKY SWEET BARBECUE SAUCE

∞

*B*arbecue sauce on pizza? Yep—try it, and you'll see. This is a delicious, fast, and easy pizza that kids as well as adults will love.

MAKES TWO 16" PIZZAS, 8 SLICES PER PIZZA

Follow pizza dough instructions on page 219.

TOPPING:

⅔ cup Smoky Sweet Barbecue Sauce (or fat-free bottled sauce)
1 cup cooked shredded skinless organic chicken breasts
¼ cup finely diced scallions

SMOKY SWEET BARBECUE SAUCE:

12-14 oz. ketchup
½ cup white vinegar
¼ cup honey
½-1 teaspoon ground chipotle, to taste
⅛ teaspoon salt

Combine all ingredients in a small saucepan and simmer stirring frequently until reduced, about 15-20 minutes. Make about 1½ cups sauce.

Preheat oven to 450°F. Brush dough very lightly with olive oil. Bake untopped dough for 5–7 minutes or until it is dry but not browning. Remove from oven, spread evenly with barbecue sauce and sprinkle with chicken and scallions. Bake for another 5–7 minutes or until edges are crispy and lightly browned.

NUTRIENT ANALYSIS PER SLICE:

Calories (kcal) 138.69

Protein (g) 6.44	Calories from Protein 26.35	% Calories from Protein 19.00
Carbohydrates (g) 25.58	Calories from Carbohydrates 104.58	% Calories from Carbohydrates 75.41
Fat (g) 0.84	Calories from Fat 7.76	% Calories from Fat 5.59
Saturated Fat (g) 0.17	Cholesterol (mg) 7.44	Total Dietary Fiber (g) 1.17
Sodium (mg) 383.30		

CRISPY PIZZA WITH WILD MUSHROOMS AND ROSEMARY

∞

*H*ere's a sophisticated pizza, if there is such a thing, that has an incredible earthy flavor and aroma.

MAKES TWO 16" PIZZAS, 8 SLICES PER PIZZA

Follow pizza dough instructions on page 219.

TOPPING:

1 tablespoon olive oil
4 cups assorted wild mushrooms
1 tablespoon rosemary

Preheat oven to 450°F. In a large non-stick skillet heat oil over medium high heat. Add mushrooms and sauté until tender and liquid has evaporated.

Brush dough very lightly with olive oil. Bake untopped dough for 5–7 minutes or until it is dry but not browning. Remove from oven, sprinkle evenly with cooked mushrooms and rosemary, and bake for another 5–7 minutes or until edges are crispy and lightly browned.

NUTRIENT ANALYSIS PER SLICE:
Calories (kcal) 127.80

Protein (g) 3.88	Calories from Protein 15.67	% Calories from Protein 12.26
Carbohydrates (g) 24.95	Calories from Carbohydrates 100.70	% Calories from Carbohydrates 78.80
Fat (g) 1.26	Calories from Fat 11.43	% Calories from Fat 8.94
Saturated Fat (g) 0.18	Total Dietary Fiber (g) 1.21	Sodium (mg) 292.39

DESSERTS

∞

ONE OF MY favorite sayings is "Life's too short. Eat dessert first." For the sake of overall good health I don't take this literally, but I am quite grateful that sugar is not an IBS trigger (it contains no insoluble fiber, no fat, no caffeine, no alcohol, and has no stimulant or irritant effect on the GI tract whatsoever). While I do try not to eat desserts with reckless abandon, I have to admit it's a struggle, as it is just so fast and easy to safely modify sweet recipes. The most common triggers in desserts are dairy and fats, and simple substitutions of egg whites for whole eggs, cocoa powder for solid chocolate, soy or rice milk for dairy, and a reduction in butter or oil is all that's needed to create luscious desserts that are perfectly tolerable for IBS.

So go ahead and enjoy delicious homestyle favorites like Old-Fashioned Banana Creme Pie, Chocolate Chip Peppermint Ice Dream Sandwiches, Double Decker Sweet Potato Pecan Pie, and Brer Rabbit Carrot Cake, as well as more exotic sweet treats such as Sultry Summer Mango Sorbet, Mandarin Chocolate Sponge Cake, or Cinnamon Walnut Tart with Raspberry Sauce. The sky really is the limit when it comes to safe, scrumptious dessert choices, so feel free to indulge occasionally.

BETTER THAN CHEESECAKE
∞

VARIATIONS: SUMMER FRUIT TOPPING
AND SWEET-TART LEMON CURD TOPPING

*W*hy is it better? Because unlike the real thing, this cheesecake won't trigger an attack. Silky smooth and subtly sweet, this dessert has the ethereal texture of a light and creamy mousse. It is more luscious than you could ever imagine. I make it all summer long with different fresh fruit toppings, and have been known to eat it for breakfast when no one's looking. If you serve this to company without mentioning the tofu, I guarantee you'll be asked for the recipe.

MAKES ONE 10" CAKE—14-16 SERVINGS

CRUST:

8 graham crackers, finely crushed
1 tablespoon canola oil

Preheat oven to 325°F. Lightly spray 10" non-stick heavy-gauge springform pan with cooking oil. Mix all crust ingredients together thoroughly and press firmly into pan. Bake 4–5 mins. Cool on rack.

FILLING:

Two 12.3 oz. packages Mori-Nu Silken Firm tofu, the "light" version if possible
⅓ cup fresh lemon (or lime or orange juice)*
Grated rind from 2 lemons (or 4 limes or 1 orange)*
4 organic egg whites
3 tablespoons cornstarch
⅔—¾ cup granulated sugar, to taste

Raise oven temperature to 350°F. Mix all ingredients together in blender at high speed until thoroughly combined. Do not use mixer, as recipe will not work using it. You may have to carefully scrape down sides of blender with a rubber spatula while the motor is running. Slowly pour filling into cooled crust. Bake at 350°F. for 20–25 minutes. Pie will not look set in middle. Cool on rack and chill several hours or overnight in pan. Carefully spread with fruit topping or lemon curd (optional). Chill until topping is set. Run a long thin knife around edge of pan and carefully remove sides. Serve chilled.

*Lemon really tastes the best

Nutrient Analysis Per Serving Without Topping:
Calories (kcal) 101.18

Protein (g) 4.18	Calories from Protein 16.47	% Calories from Protein 16.27
Carbohydrates (g) 17.12	Calories from Carbohydrates 67.52	% Calories from Carbohydrates 66.74
Fat (g) 1.94	Calories from Fat 17.19	% Calories from Fat 16.99
Saturated Fat (g) 0.23	Total Dietary Fiber (g) 0.23	Sodium (mg) 93.98

Summer Fruit Topping:

Makes 1 topping for 10" cheesecake

2 cups fresh blueberries, pitted cherries, skinned/chopped apricots or peaches,
   or raspberries
½ cup fresh lemon or orange juice
¼ cup granulated sugar plus 2 tablespoons cornstarch, stirred together

Bring fruit and juice to a boil in saucepan or microwave. Simmer for 2–3 minutes.
Berries should pop; other fruit should start to disintegrate. Remove from heat and stir
in sugar/cornstarch mixture. Fruit should thicken as you stir without further cooking.
Spread over cooled cheesecake and chill until cold.

Sweet-Tart Lemon Curd Topping:

Makes 1 topping for 10" cheesecake

1 cup granulated sugar
3 tablespoons cornstarch
2 teaspoons all-purpose unbleached white flour
Dash salt
1 cup boiling water
4 teaspoons grated lemon zest
6 tablespoons fresh lemon juice
1 tablespoon soy cream cheese or soy sour cream

In a large saucepan whisk together the sugar, cornstarch, flour, and salt.

In a medium bowl whisk together the water, zest, and juice.

Whisk the liquid into the saucepan thoroughly, using a rubber spatula to scrape around
sides and bottom. Place pan over medium heat and whisk constantly until mixture boils.
Whisk for one full minute (mixture should thicken and turn clear). Remove from heat.

Microwave cream cheese for a few seconds until softened. Whisk into curd thoroughly.
Spread curd over cooled cheesecake. Refrigerate until cold (curd will thicken as it cools).

BANANA BUTTERSCOTCH SOUFFLÉS

∞

hese make a spectacular presentation for a formal dessert. The soufflés rise high and golden above their bowls, and inside they are creamy, sweet, and rich. Oh, and did I mention they're almost fat free and full of soluble fiber, too? Enjoy.

MAKES 4 SERVINGS

> 3 large organic egg whites
> ¼ cup granulated sugar
> 2 firm-ripe bananas
> 2 tablespoons butterscotch chips, finely chopped

Preheat oven to 450°F and spray four 2–cup capacity ramekins or bowls with cooking oil. In a large bowl beat egg whites until they hold soft peaks and gradually beat in sugar until egg whites hold stiff peaks. Coarsely grate the bananas into the meringue and fold in with the butterscotch chips.

Place ramekins on a cookie sheet and fill with batter, mounding it in the centers of the ramekins and running a knife along the sides of ramekins after they have been filled with batter to aid rising. Bake in center of oven for 15 minutes, or until puffed and golden brown. Serve immediately (soufflés will deflate quickly).

NUTRIENT ANALYSIS PER SERVING:
Calories (kcal) 126.03

Protein (g) 3.46	Calories from Protein 12.89	% Calories from Protein 10.23
Carbohydrates (g) 26.21	Calories from Carbohydrates 97.57	% Calories from Carbohydrates 77.42
Fat (g) 1.86	Calories from Fat 15.56	% Calories from Fat 12.35
Saturated Fat (g) 1.04	Total Dietary Fiber (g) 1.73	Sodium (mg) 45.78

TAHITIAN VANILLA BEAN PUDDING
∞

VARIATIONS: TAHITIAN VANILLA BEAN CUSTARD
PIE AND TAHITIAN VANILLA BEAN ICE CREAM

It's hard to imagine a more soothing food than vanilla pudding. This is the stuff childhood memories are made of—sweet, creamy, and rich.

MAKES 6 SERVINGS

½ large fresh Tahitian vanilla bean
3 cups vanilla soy or rice milk
6 tablespoons granulated sugar
6 tablespoons cornstarch
Dash salt
6 tablespoons corn syrup
3 organic egg whites

Working over a small saucepan, slit vanilla bean and scrape out seeds, adding pod and seeds to the saucepan. Add the milk and bring to a boil, whisking. Remove from heat and let cool. Remove and discard pod, scraping any remaining seeds into milk.

In a small bowl beat the egg whites until lightly frothy. Set aside.

In a heavy, large double boiler whisk together sugar, cornstarch, and salt. Gradually whisk in the cooled vanilla milk and corn syrup, and scrape around the bottom and edges of the pan with a rubber spatula until thoroughly blended. Set pan over boiling water and cook, whisking constantly until the mixture reaches a full boil. Continue whisking for one more minute, and remove from heat.

Carefully whisk several large spoonfuls of hot pudding into the egg whites to temper them. Add the egg mixture back to the pan of pudding and whisk well to thoroughly blend.

Return the pan to the heat and whisk constantly for one minute until mixture thickens. Pour into six serving glasses and chill until cold.

Variations: Pudding may also be used as pie filling with a graham cracker crust or frozen in an ice cream maker according to manufacturer's directions.

NUTRIENT ANALYSIS PER SERVING:
Calories (kcal) 169.50

Protein (g) 5.15	Calories from Protein 19.74	% Calories from Protein 11.65
Carbohydrates (g) 33.77	Calories from Carbohydrates 129.53	% Calories from Carbohydrates 76.42
Fat (g) 2.34	Calories from Fat 20.23	% Calories from Fat 11.93
Saturated Fat (g) 0.26	Total Dietary Fiber (g) 1.66	Sodium (mg) 70.52

CHOCOLATE SILK PUDDING

∞

VARIATIONS: CHOCOLATE SILK PIE
AND CHOCOLATE SILK ICE CREAM

This recipe makes what is undoubtedly the richest pudding I have ever tasted. It is hard to believe that it is virtually fat-free. I grew up on homemade puddings and missed them dearly when IBS made it impossible for me to keep eating them. Fortunately, when I discovered soy milk, I could once again eat pudding to my heart's content. So I do!

When frozen as ice cream this pudding is almost too rich—so dense, fudgy, and creamy it will put even a die-hard chocoholic into a euphoric haze.

MAKES 6 SERVINGS

> 6 tablespoons granulated sugar
> ½ cup unsweetened cocoa powder
> 6 tablespoons cornstarch
> Dash salt
> 3 cups vanilla soy or rice milk
> 6 tablespoons corn syrup
> 3 organic egg whites
> I tablespoon vanilla extract
> ½ teaspoon almond extract (optional)

In a small bowl beat the egg whites until lightly frothy. Set aside.

In a heavy, large double boiler whisk together first four ingredients. Gradually whisk in the milk and corn syrup, and scrape around the bottom and edges of the pan with a rubber spatula until thoroughly blended. Set pan over boiling water and cook, whisking constantly until the mixture reaches a full boil. Continue whisking for one more minute and remove from heat.

Carefully whisk several large spoonfuls of hot pudding into the egg whites to temper them. Add the egg mixture back to the pan of pudding and whisk well to thoroughly blend.

Return the pan to the heat and whisk constantly for one minute until mixture thickens. Remove from heat and whisk in vanilla (and almond) extract. Pour into six serving glasses and chill until cold.

Variations: Pudding may also be used as pie filling with a graham cracker crust or frozen in an ice cream maker according to manufacturer's directions.

NUTRIENT ANALYSIS PER SERVING:
Calories (kcal) 207.07

Protein (g) 6.55	Calories from Protein 24.32	% Calories from Protein 11.74
Carbohydrates (g) 41.76	Calories from Carbohydrates 154.98	% Calories from Carbohydrates 74.84
Fat (g) 3.33	Calories from Fat 27.78	% Calories from Fat 13.41
Saturated Fat (g) 0.84	Total Dietary Fiber (g) 4.04	Sodium (mg) 101.47

INDIAN PISTACHIO ORANGE BLOSSOM TAPIOCA PUDDING

∞

*T*his pudding is a study in contrasts—exotic with the heady perfume of orange flower water but with the comforting familiarity of old-fashioned tapioca. It is subtly spiced and makes an unusual and filling breakfast, or a lovely finish to a meal of Bengali Spiced Chickpeas, Tomatoes, and Spinach with Black Salt (page 207), pappadams, and jasmine rice.

MAKES 4-6 SERVINGS

> 2 cups water
> 1 cup uncooked tapioca
> 1 teaspoon canola oil
> 2 tablespoons chopped dates
> 2 tablespoons chopped unsalted natural (not red-dyed) pistachios
> 2 cups soy or rice milk
> ½ cup brown sugar
> ⅛ teaspoon ground cardamom
> ⅛ teaspoon ground nutmeg
> 1 tablespoon orange flower water*

Bring water to boil in a large saucepan. Add the tapioca and simmer over medium heat until tender and translucent, about 15–20 minutes. Set aside.

In a small non-stick skillet heat the oil. Add the dates and pistachios and sauté until the nuts are golden and the dates plump.

Add the dates, pistachios, milk, sugar, cardamom, and nutmeg to the tapioca. Simmer over low heat for 5 minutes. Fold in orange flower water. Serve warm or chilled.

*See **Specialty Ingredients** (page 34)

NUTRIENT ANALYSIS PER SERVING:
Calories (kcal) 234.64

Protein (g) 3.50	Calories from Protein 13.63	% Calories from Protein 5.81
Carbohydrates(g) 46.91	Calories from Carbohydrates 182.65	% Calories from Carbohydrates 77.84
Fat (g) 4.38	Calories from Fat 38.37	% Calories from Fat 16.35
Saturated Fat (g) 0.48	Total Dietary Fiber (g) 2.23	Sodium (mg) 18.04

SULTRY SUMMER MANGO SORBET

∞

*O*oh, this sorbet is so exotically luscious and has such a heady tropical perfume it will make you swoon. It is in fact a very virtuous dessert but it certainly tastes sinful. There's an added bonus here—mangoes are one of the single most nutritious foods you can eat, which means this recipe is not only safe but downright healthy.

MAKES 6-8 SERVINGS (ABOUT 1 QUART)

- 2 cups water
- ½ cup granulated sugar
- 1 tablespoon fresh lemon juice
- 4 cups pitted, diced, fresh very ripe mango (about 4 large mangoes)
- 2 organic egg whites*

In a small saucepan make a simple syrup by combining water and sugar, stirring and heating until sugar dissolves. Chill. Combine syrup with remaining ingredients in blender. Blend on high until well mixed. Freeze in ice cream maker according to manufacturer's instructions.

*If salmonella is a concern in your area you can substitute pasteurized egg whites, available in the dairy section of most grocery stores (such as Egg Beaters).

NUTRIENT ANALYSIS PER SERVING:
Calories (kcal) 142.20

Protein (g) 1.74	Calories from Protein 6.50	% Calories from Protein 4.57
Carbohydrates (g) 35.68	Calories from Carbohydrates 133.21	% Calories from Carbohydrates 93.67
Fat (g) 0.30	Calories from Fat 2.49	% Calories from Fat 1.75
Saturated Fat (g) 0.07	Total Dietary Fiber (g) 1.99	Sodium (mg) 20.65

Pucker up,
Buttercup Lemon Sorbet

∞

This sorbet is tart, sweet, refreshing, and absolutely delightful on a hot summer day. The first time I tasted this recipe I positively shivered with pleasure and my mouth puckered up from the lemons. My husband's nickname for me is Buttercup—need I say more?

MAKES 6-8 SERVINGS (ABOUT 1 QUART)

> 2 cups water
> 2 cups granulated sugar
> Juice and zest of 4 large lemons
> 2 organic egg whites*

In a small saucepan make a simple syrup by combining water and sugar, stirring and heating until sugar dissolves. Chill. Combine syrup with remaining ingredients in blender. Blend on high until well mixed. Freeze in ice cream maker according to manufacturer's instructions.

*If salmonella is a concern in your area you can substitute pasteurized egg whites, available in the dairy section of most grocery stores (such as Egg Beaters).

NUTRIENT ANALYSIS PER SERVING:
Calories (kcal) 271.40

Protein (g) 1.29	Calories from Protein 4.95	% Calories from Protein 1.83
Carbohydrates (g) 69.42	Calories from Carbohydrates 266.45	% Calories from Carbohydrates 98.17
Total Dietary Fiber (g) 0.13	Sodium (mg) 19.24	

FRESH MINT LEAF AND LIME SORBET

∞

*T*his is a very elegant and delicious sorbet that is a lovely pastel shade of cool green. It makes a wonderful finale to any Thai or Mexican meal. For a formal dessert presentation, serve individual scoops in tall crystal glasses garnished with an extra mint leaf or two.

MAKES 6-8 SERVINGS (ABOUT 1 QUART)

2 cups water
2 cups granulated sugar
3 cups packed fresh mint leaves, washed, dried, and chopped
1 cup fresh lime juice
1 tablespoon grated lime zest
2 organic egg whites*

Make a mint syrup by combining mint leaves, sugar, and water in a small saucepan. Heat and stir until sugar dissolves, bring to a boil and simmer 2 minutes. Chill. Strain syrup, pressing hard on solids and discarding mint leaves. Add syrup and remaining ingredients in blender, mixing well on high speed. Freeze in ice cream maker according to manufacturer's instructions.

*If salmonella is a concern in your area you can substitute pasteurized egg whites, available in the dairy section of most grocery stores (such as Egg Beaters).

NUTRIENT ANALYSIS PER SERVING:
Calories (kcal) 274.64

Protein (g) 1.35	Calories from Protein 5.17	% Calories from Protein 1.88
Carbohydrates (g) 70.41	Calories from Carbohydrates 269.12	% Calories from Carbohydrates 97.99
Fat (g) 0.04	Calories from Fat 0.35	% Calories from Fat 0.13
Saturated Fat (g) 0.00	Total Dietary Fiber (g) 0.16	Sodium (mg) 19.34

FLORENTINE PEACH GELATO
∞

*P*eaches are my favorite summer fruit, and this gelato is one of the most delicious ways to eat them. Bring a quart of this to your next backyard barbecue and pity the people eating ice cream.

MAKES 6-8 SERVINGS (ABOUT I QUART)

I cup granulated sugar
½ cup plus I tablespoon water
2 cups finely diced and peeled fresh ripe peaches
2 tablespoons fresh lemon juice
I organic egg white*

Combine sugar and water in a small saucepan and heat until sugar dissolves. Cool syrup. Purée peaches with syrup, lemon juice, and egg white in a blender or food processor until completely smooth. Freeze in ice cream maker according to manufacturer's instructions.

*If salmonella is a concern in your area you can substitute pasteurized egg whites, available in the dairy section of most grocery stores (such as Egg Beaters).

NUTRIENT ANALYSIS PER SERVING:
Calories (kcal) 157.42

Protein (g) 1.00	Calories from Protein 3.83	% Calories from Protein 2.43
Carbohydrates (g) 40.09	Calories from Carbohydrates 153.16	% Calories from Carbohydrates 97.29
Fat (g) 0.05	Calories from Fat 0.44	% Calories from Fat 0.28
Saturated Fat (g) 0.01	Total Dietary Fiber (g) 1.15	Sodium (mg) 9.51

FRESH TANGERINE GELATO

∞

*T*his gelato has a bright, fresh flavor that is irresistible. It makes a wonderful light dessert to virtually any meal, but is especially welcome after Mexican food.

MAKES 6-8 SERVINGS (ABOUT 1 QUART)

7 cups fresh tangerine juice
1½ cups granulated sugar
2 organic egg whites*

Stir together juice and sugar until sugar dissolves. Whip in blender with egg whites until smooth. Freeze in ice cream maker according to manufacturer's instructions.

*If salmonella is a concern in your area you can substitute pasteurized egg whites, available in the dairy section of most grocery stores (such as Egg Beaters).

NUTRIENT ANALYSIS PER SERVING:
Calories (kcal) 322.98

Protein (g) 2.61	Calories from Protein 10.16	% Calories from Protein 3.14
Carbohydrates (g) 79.17	Calories from Carbohydrates 307.78	% Calories from Carbohydrates 95.29
Fat (g) 0.58	Calories from Fat 5.04	% Calories from Fat 1.56
Saturated Fat (g) 0.07	Total Dietary Fiber (g) 0.58	Sodium (mg) 21.64

CHOCOLATE CHIP PEPPERMINT ICE DREAM SANDWICHES

*T*hink you can't eat ice cream? You can eat these—the mint chocolate chip ice cream cookies of your childhood dreams! They are surprisingly easy to make and fun to assemble. They're the perfect treat for a casual summer dessert or a child's birthday party. If you can tolerate solid chocolate, the optional chocolate chips add the perfect touch.

MAKES ABOUT 12 SANDWICHES

PEPPERMINT ICE DREAM:

MAKES 3½ CUPS

  ½ cup granulated sugar
  1 tablespoon cornstarch
  2⅓ cups unsweetened soy milk
  2 organic egg whites, beaten lightly
  2 tablespoons green Crème de Menthe*
  ¼ teaspoon peppermint extract
  2 tablespoons semi-sweet chocolate—not unsweetened—finely chopped or
    grated

In a large saucepan whisk together sugar and cornstarch, then whisk in soy milk. Bring to a boil over medium heat, whisking frequently, and boil whisking constantly for one minute. Remove from heat. Whisk several large spoonfuls of hot milk mixture into egg whites, then whisk egg mixture back into saucepan of hot milk. Return saucepan to heat and cook over medium flame, whisking constantly, until mixture returns to a boil. Transfer mixture to a bowl and refrigerate until cold. Freeze mixture in ice cream maker according to manufacturer's directions. (Add chopped chocolate towards the end of the freezing process.)

*Clear Crème de Menthe can be substituted, but it won't add the pretty green color

CHOCOLATE COOKIE SANDWICHES:

MAKES 24 COOKIES

    I cup all-purpose unbleached white flour
    I cup granulated sugar
    ½ cup unsweetened cocoa powder
    I teaspoon baking powder
    ½ teaspoon salt
    ¼ cup canola oil
    4 organic egg whites, lightly beaten

Sift first 5 ingredients into a large bowl, and whisk together until thoroughly combined. In a small bowl whisk together oil and egg whites, then add liquid mixture to dry and stir until well-combined. Cover dough and refrigerate until firm, 1–2 hours.

Preheat oven to 400°F. Spray 2 large cookie sheets with cooking oil. Roll generous tablespoonfulls of dough into balls and arrange, evenly spaced, on cookie sheets (cookies will not spread). Flatten each ball with your hand (dampen hands with cold water first) until ¼" thick. Bake 8–9 minutes until set but not hard. Do not overbake. Immediately transfer cookies to rack to cool.

To Assemble Sandwiches: soften peppermint ice dream slightly. Spread a generous amount of ice dream between two cookies (filling should be twice as thick as cookies), pressing sandwich together very gently. Set sandwiches on a cookie sheet, uncovered, and freeze until firm. When hard, wrap each cookie individually in plastic wrap.

NUTRIENT ANALYSIS PER SANDWICH:
Calories (kcal) 229.71

Protein (g) 4.92	Calories from Protein 19.19	% Calories from Protein 8.36
Carbohydrates (g) 38.89	Calories from Carbohydrates 151.69	% Calories from Carbohydrates 66.03
Fat (g) 6.70	Calories from Fat 58.83	% Calories from Fat 25.61
Saturated Fat (g) 1.05	Total Dietary Fiber (g) 2.20	Sodium (mg) 172.24

SWEET MOROCCAN JEWELED COUSCOUS

∞

*T*his dessert is almost a pudding but not quite. It's unusually delicious, quite lovely, and is a very festive dessert to serve to guests. It's just subtly sweet and makes a nice change of pace for breakfast. The couscous gives a safe soluble fiber base to the nuts and dried fruit; overall this is one of the most nutritious desserts imaginable.

MAKES 6-8 SERVINGS

1 ⅓ cups couscous
2 cups water
1 tablespoon canola oil
⅓ cup granulated sugar
1 ¼ cups vanilla soy or rice milk
½ cup finely chopped dates
¼ cup finely chopped golden raisins
¼ cup finely chopped dried cherries
½ cup shelled and chopped unsalted, natural (not dyed-red) pistachios

Bring water to a boil in microwave, add couscous, and cover. Let sit for 5 minutes. Uncover and fluff with a fork. Drizzle in oil and sugar, and stir well. Add all remaining ingredients and gently combine. Serve warm or cold.

NUTRIENT ANALYSIS PER SERVING:
Calories (kcal) 274.94

Protein (g) 6.41	Calories from Protein 24.83	% Calories from Protein 9.03
Carbohydrates (g) 48.88	Calories from Carbohydrates 189.25	% Calories from Carbohydrates 68.83
Fat (g) 6.99	Calories from Fat 60.86	% Calories from Fat 22.14
Saturated Fat (g) 0.81	Total Dietary Fiber (g) 4.13	Sodium (mg) 10.19

MELTAWAY RASPBERRY ANGEL KISSES

∞

VARIATIONS: CHOCOLATE KISSES

*T*he lightest, airiest, most guilt-free cookies imaginable—and you could eat the whole batch without fear of triggering an attack. The raspberry kisses are a delicate pale pink, while the chocolate ones have luscious streaks of cocoa. Make both for Valentine's Day and share them with your sweetie.

MAKES ABOUT 36 COOKIES

3 organic egg whites, at room temperature
¼ teaspoon cream of tartar
⅛ teaspoon salt
¾ cup granulated sugar
¼ cup seedless red raspberry preserves
7–8 drops red food coloring if desired

Preheat oven to 250°F. Cover 2 cookie sheets with parchment paper or brown paper (from brown paper bags). In large bowl, beat egg whites, cream of tartar, and salt until soft peaks form. Gradually add sugar, beating until very stiff peaks form, about 5 minutes. Add preserves (and food coloring) and beat one minute at high speed. Drop meringue by small teaspoonfuls or pipe with pastry tube into one-inch mounds onto lined cookie sheets. Bake for 40–45 minutes, or until the tops of cookies feel dry to the touch. Reduce heat if they begin to brown. Cool completely before removing from paper.

FOR CHOCOLATE KISSES:

Omit raspberry preserves and food coloring. Fold 2 tablespoons unsweetened cocoa powder into the finished meringue. Continue as directed above.

NUTRIENT ANALYSIS PER COOKIE:
Calories (kcal) 22.95

Protein (g) 0.31	Calories from Protein 1.19	% Calories from Protein 5.18
Carbohydrates (g) 5.64	Calories from Carbohydrates 21.72	% Calories from Carbohydrates 94.65
Fat (g) 0.00	Calories from Fat 0.04	% Calories from Fat 0.17
Saturated Fat (g) 0.00	Total Dietary Fiber (g) 0.02	Sodium (mg) 13.58

BRER RABBIT CARROT CAKE

I love traditional carrot cake oh-so-much, but for reasons I've never been able to fathom most recipes are typically very high in oil. There is no need for that with this version, as the shredded carrots and crushed pineapple make the cake deliciously and virtuously moist. It is scrumptious served plain, or you can add the icing for a touch of sweet decadence.

MAKES 16 SERVINGS

Preheat oven to 350°F. Spray a 10" non-stick bundt pan with cooking oil and set aside. Sift into a large bowl and stir well to combine:

1½ cups all-purpose unbleached white flour
1½ teaspoons baking powder
¾ teaspoon baking soda
2 teaspoons cinnamon
½ teaspoon allspice
½ teaspoon nutmeg
¾ cup granulated sugar

In a separate large bowl beat with an electric mixer until well combined:

¼ cup packed brown sugar
¾ cup organic egg whites
½ cup canola oil
2 tablespoons fresh orange zest
1 teaspoon vanilla
1½–2 cups packed finely shredded or grated carrots
¾ cup canned crushed pineapple, with liquid

Add the wet ingredients to the dry with just a few swift strokes by hand. Do not over-beat or the cake will be tough. Pour batter into prepared pan and bake for 45–55 minutes, until toothpick or cake tester inserted into center comes out clean. Cool on rack for 10 minutes, then invert onto rack and cool to room temperature. Top with Sweet Orange Icing (do not top while cake is still warm).

SWEET ORANGE ICING:

¾ cup sifted confectioners' sugar
1½ teaspoons fresh orange zest
1 tablespoons fresh orange juice
½ teaspoon fresh lemon juice

Combine all ingredients and blend with a fork until smooth. Use immediately to top cake (if icing sits it will harden).

NUTRIENT ANALYSIS PER SERVING:
Calories (kcal) 169.45

Protein (g) 2.56	Calories from Protein 10.11	% Calories from Protein 5.97
Carbohydrates (g) 24.77	Calories from Carbohydrates 97.64	% Calories from Carbohydrates 57.62
Fat (g) 6.96	Calories from Fat 61.70	% Calories from Fat 36.41
Saturated Fat (g) 0.51	Total Dietary Fiber (g) 0.72	Sodium (mg) 128.78

OLD-FASHIONED BANANA CREME PIE

VARIATIONS: CHOCOLATE AND PUDDING

*W*ho could resist? Everyone loves traditional, homemade creme pies, and luckily it's a snap to make perfectly safe versions. This dessert is low fat, non-dairy, and has high soluble fiber—but it tastes so rich and delicious you'll be too busy enjoying it to care.

MAKES A 9" PIE, 8 SERVINGS

CRUST:

8 graham crackers, finely crushed
I tablespoon canola oil

Preheat oven to 325°F. Lightly spray 9" Pyrex pie pan with cooking oil. Mix all crust ingredients together thoroughly and press firmly into pan. Bake 4–5 mins. Cool on rack.

FILLING:

2 firm-ripe bananas
⅓ cup brown sugar
½ cup all-purpose unbleached white flour
½ teaspoon salt
2 cups vanilla soy milk
5 organic egg whites, lightly beaten until frothy
I tablespoon vanilla

Thinly slice bananas onto baked pie crust and set aside. In a large heavy double boiler whisk together sugar, flour, and salt. Whisk in milk, scraping around sides with a rubber spatula as necessary, and set pan over boiling water. Cook until mixture thickens, about 10 minutes, whisking constantly. Remove from heat and carefully whisk several large spoonfuls of hot pudding into the egg whites to temper them. Add the egg mixture back to the pan of pudding and whisk well to thoroughly blend.

Return the pan to the heat and whisk constantly until thickened. Remove from heat and add vanilla. Pour pudding over bananas into crust. Smooth top and chill.

CHOCOLATE VARIATION FOR CRUST:

Add 1 tablespoon unsweetened cocoa powder to crust ingredients before baking

CHOCOLATE VARIATION FOR FILLING:

Add ⅓ cup unsweetened cocoa powder and 1 tablespoon granulated sugar to dry ingredients

PUDDING VARIATION:

Omit crust. Fold sliced bananas into cooked pudding mixture and spoon into 8 decorative glasses. Chill.

NUTRIENT ANALYSIS PER SERVING:
Calories (kcal) 183.63

Protein (g) 5.96	Calories from Protein 23.26	% Calories from Protein 12.67
Carbohydrates(g) 30.83	Calories from Carbohydrates 120.38	% Calories from Carbohydrates 65.55
Fat (g) 4.55	Calories from Fat 39.99	% Calories from Fat 21.78
Saturated Fat (g) 0.53	Total Dietary Fiber (g) 2.11	Sodium (mg) 274.44

PEPPERMINT FUDGE CAKE
∞

*T*his recipe is sinfully rich with deep dark chocolate, incredibly easy to make, and completely safe to eat. Children love the peppermint, and it's a sure-fire hit at parties. For a delicious alternative try the almond variation. This cake freezes beautifully unfrosted, and travels well, too. I have shipped it to family and friends for Christmas.

MAKES 12 SERVINGS

Preheat oven to 325°F. Spray a 10" non-stick bundt pan with cooking oil and set aside. Sift together in large bowl and stir together well:

2 cups all-purpose unbleached white flour
2 teaspoons baking soda
6 tablespoons unsweetened cocoa powder
1 tablespoon cornstarch
1 cup granulated sugar
½ teaspoon salt

Stir together by hand in medium bowl:

1¾ cup unsweetened applesauce, homemade (page 78) or bottled
¼ cup canola oil
1 tablespoon vanilla
1 tablespoon peppermint extract

Add the wet ingredients to the dry with a few swift strokes just until blended. Pour into bundt pan. Bake 50–60 minutes. Cool on rack. Top with Mocha Mint Glaze (do not top while cake is still warm).

MOCHA MINT GLAZE:

½ cup confectioners' sugar
2 tablespoons unsweetened cocoa powder
½ teaspoon decaffeinated instant coffee powder
1½ tablespoons water or soy or rice milk
½ teaspoon peppermint extract

Sift sugar and cocoa into medium bowl. Dissolve coffee in 1 tablespoon of the water or milk and add the mint extract. Gradually whisk coffee liquid into dry ingredients. Whisk in additional ½ tablespoon of water or milk if necessary. Use glaze immediately to top bundt cake (if glaze sits it will harden).

Variation: For a lovely alternative, substitute 1 tablespoon almond extract for the peppermint extract in the cake, and replace the ½ teaspoon peppermint extract in the icing with ½ teaspoon almond extract.

NUTRIENT ANALYSIS PER SERVING WITHOUT GLAZE:
Calories (kcal) 205.61

Protein (g) 2.74	Calories from Protein 10.60	% Calories from Protein 5.16
Carbohydrates(g) 38.64	Calories from Carbohydrates 149.29	% Calories from Carbohydrates 72.61
Fat (g) 5.26	Calories from Fat 45.72	% Calories from Fat 22.24
Saturated Fat (g) 0.58	Total Dietary Fiber (g) 1.89	Sodium (mg) 308.58

MANDARIN CHOCOLATE SPONGE CAKE WITH SWEET ORANGE ICING

∞

*T*his cake is light, sophisticated, and has a classic orange-chocolate flavor combination.

MAKES 12 SERVINGS

Preheat oven to 350°F. Spray a 10" non-stick bundt pan with cooking oil and set aside. Sift into a large bowl and stir together well:

2½ cups all-purpose unbleached white flour

2 cups powdered sugar

½ cup unsweetened cocoa powder

1¾ teaspoons baking powder

½ teaspoon baking soda

Dash salt

In another large bowl beat with an electric mixer until well combined:

1⅓ cups brown sugar

⅔ cup canola oil

1 cup organic egg whites (from about 10 eggs)

1¼ cups soy or rice milk

½ cup fresh orange juice

1 tablespoon vanilla extract

1 teaspoon orange oil

1 tablespoon orange zest

Pour the wet ingredients into the dry and mix with a few swift strokes until just blended. Do not overbeat or the cake will be tough. Pour the batter into the prepared pan and bake for 45–50 minutes, until a toothpick or cake tester inserted into the center of the cake comes out clean. Cool on rack in pan for 20 minutes, then invert cake and cool on plate to room temperature. Top with Sweet Orange Icing (do not top cake until it has cooled).

Sweet Orange Icing:

1½ cups sifted confectioners' sugar
1 tablespoon fresh orange zest
2 tablespoons fresh orange juice
1 teaspoon fresh lemon juice

Combine all ingredients and blend with a fork until smooth. Use immediately to top cake (icing will harden if it sits).

NUTRIENT ANALYSIS PER SERVING WITHOUT ICING:
Calories (kcal) 375.33

Protein (g) 6.30	Calories from Protein 24.47	% Calories from Protein 6.52
Carbohydrates (g) 59.33	Calories from Carbohydrates 230.53	% Calories from Carbohydrates 61.42
Fat (g) 13.76	Calories from Fat 120.33	% Calories from Fat 32.06
Saturated Fat (g) 1.27	Total Dietary Fiber (g) 2.25	Sodium (mg) 167.68

CHOCOLATE PECAN FALLEN SOUFFLÉ CAKE WITH RASPBERRY SAUCE

∞

*T*his cake is so dense and fudgy it's almost a torte. It's delicious plain but truly decadent with the raspberry sauce. This recipe is a perfect example of how tolerable nuts can be when finely ground.

MAKES 12 SERVINGS

⅔ cup pecans, finely ground
½ cup unsweetened cocoa powder
1 tablespoon decaffeinated instant coffee granules (optional)
1½ cups granulated sugar
7 large organic egg whites
¼ teaspoon salt
3 tablespoons canola oil
1 teaspoon vanilla

Preheat oven to 350°F. Spray a 9" non-stick springform pan with cooking spray and set aside. In a medium bowl whisk together ground pecans, cocoa, coffee granules, and ¾ cup sugar.

In a large bowl beat egg whites with salt until they hold soft peaks. Gradually add remaining ¾ cup sugar while continuing to beat mixture, then whip until it just holds stiff peaks. Gently fold one third of egg white mixture into pecan mixture to lighten the batter. Partially fold remaining egg white mixture into pecans, then add oil and vanilla and fold all ingredients together gently but thoroughly.

Pour batter into prepared pan, smooth top, and bake 35–40 minutes or until a tester inserted in middle comes out with moist crumbs. Immediately run a thin sharp knife around edges of cake to loosen from the sides of the pan, then cool cake, in the pan, on a rack (it will fall as it cools). Run a thin knife around edge of pan again and remove side of pan. Slice with a thin sharp knife and serve with raspberry sauce.

RASPBERRY SAUCE:

10 oz. package frozen sweetened raspberries
2 teaspoons cornstarch
1 teaspoon fresh lemon juice

Drain raspberries, reserving liquid. Combine liquid and cornstarch. In a small saucepan cook cornstarch liquid over medium heat, stirring constantly, until it boils. Add berries and lemon juice and cook one minute. Serve warm.

NUTRIENT ANALYSIS PER SERVING WITHOUT SAUCE:
Calories (kcal) 189.73

Protein (g) 3.26	Calories from Protein 12.23	% Calories from Protein 6.45
Carbohydrates (g) 28.33	Calories from Carbohydrates 106.15	% Calories from Carbohydrates 55.95
Fat (g) 8.46	Calories from Fat 71.35	% Calories from Fat 37.61
Saturated Fat (g) 0.90	Total Dietary Fiber (g) 1.69	Sodium (mg) 81.47

PUMPKIN SPICE PIE
WITH PRALINE TOPPING

∞

This is one of my traditional holiday dessert recipes. It's great without the topping too, but I prefer to gild the lily. That's what desserts are for!

MAKES 12-14 SERVINGS

CRUST:

8 graham crackers, finely crushed
1 tablespoon canola oil

Preheat oven to 325°F. Lightly spray 10" non-stick heavy-gauge springform pan with cooking oil. Mix all crust ingredients together thoroughly and press firmly into pan. Bake 4–5 mins. Cool on rack.

FILLING:

1½ 12.3oz. packages Mori-Nu Lite Firm tofu
2 cups canned or cooked pumpkin
⅓ cup brown sugar
⅓ cup honey
2 teaspoons cinnamon
1 teaspoon ground ginger
½ teaspoon nutmeg
¼ teaspoon cloves
¼ teaspoon salt

Raise oven temperature to 350°F. Add all filling ingredients to blender and purée until smooth, scraping down sides with rubber spatula as necessary. Carefully pour filling into cooled baked pie crust and bake for about 1 hour. Pie will appear soft in middle but will set as it cools. Allow pie to cool to room temperature. Sprinkle evenly with Praline Pecan Topping and place under broiler until topping bubbles, watching closely so it doesn't burn. Chill pie overnight before slicing.

PRALINE TOPPING:

⅓ cup packed brown sugar
½ cup finely chopped pecans
2 tablespoons canola oil

Combine all topping ingredients in small bowl, stirring well.

NUTRIENT ANALYSIS PER SERVING:
Calories (kcal) 192.03

Protein (g) 4.18	Calories from Protein 16.01	% Calories from Protein 8.34
Carbohydrates (g) 27.44	Calories from Carbohydrates 104.98	% Calories from Carbohydrates 54.67
Fat (g) 8.25	Calories from Fat 71.03	% Calories from Fat 36.99
Saturated Fat (g) 0.78	Total Dietary Fiber (g) 1.84	Sodium (mg) 146.67

DOUBLE DECKER
SWEET POTATO PECAN PIE

This is quite possibly the most delicious sweet potato pie and the best pecan pie ever—all rolled into one. It is also low fat, full of soluble fiber and nutrients, and a fabulously rich and decadent dessert that is perfectly safe to eat. In my house it just isn't Thanksgiving without a slice of Double Decker Sweet Potato Pecan Pie.

MAKES 14-16 SERVINGS

CRUST:

8 graham crackers, finely crushed
1 tablespoon canola oil

Preheat oven to 325°F. Lightly spray 10" non-stick heavy-gauge springform pan with cooking oil. Mix all crust ingredients together thoroughly and press firmly into pan. Bake 4–5 mins. Cool on rack.

SWEET POTATO FILLING:

2½ cups steamed sweet potatoes, mashed until smooth
1½ cups soy milk
¼ cup brown sugar
½ cup granulated sugar
¼ teaspoon salt
1 teaspoon cinnamon
½ teaspoon ground ginger
¼ teaspoon ground nutmeg
⅛ teaspoon ground cloves
4 organic egg whites

Raise oven temperature to 350°F. In a large bowl mix all ingredients until well blended and completely smooth. Set aside.

Pecan Filling:

6 organic egg whites
½ cup granulated sugar
½ teaspoon salt
2 tablespoons canola oil
1½ cups light corn syrup
1 cup finely chopped fresh pecan halves
1 tablespoon vanilla extract

Combine first 5 ingredients in large bowl and beat thoroughly until well combined. Stir in pecans and vanilla.

Pour sweet potato filling into baked pie crust and smooth top. Carefully pour pecan filling on top. Bake for 1 hour to 1 hour and 15 minutes, until a knife inserted into the pie comes out clean. Cool on rack.

NUTRIENT ANALYSIS PER SERVING:
Calories (kcal) 317.86

Protein (g) 4.73	Calories from Protein 18.14	% Calories from Protein 5.71
Carbohydrates (g) 58.05	Calories from Carbohydrates 222.50	% Calories from Carbohydrates 70.00
Fat (g) 8.96	Calories from Fat 77.22	% Calories from Fat 24.29
Saturated Fat (g) 0.78	Total Dietary Fiber (g) 1.98	Sodium (mg) 233.30

VERMONT MAPLE PIE

∞

*F*or a rich, sweet, gooey slice of maple heaven you just can't beat this pie. Maple syrup is one of my favorite New England ingredients, and this pie has got to be the all-time most delicious way to use it. If you like maple leaf sugar candy this pie will be your new favorite dessert.

MAKES A 9" PIE, 10 SERVINGS

CRUST:

8 graham crackers, finely crushed
2 tablespoon canola oil

Preheat oven to 325 °F. Lightly spray 9" heavy pie plate with cooking oil. Mix graham crackers and oil together thoroughly and press firmly into pan. Bake 4–5 mins. Cool on rack.

FILLING:

1⅔ cups packed brown sugar
4 large organic egg whites
½ cup vanilla soy milk
⅓ cup pure maple syrup, preferably dark amber
1 tablespoon canola oil
1 teaspoon vanilla
¼ teaspoon salt

Raise oven temperature to 350°F. In a medium bowl whisk together sugar and egg whites until creamy. Add remaining ingredients and whisk well until smooth. Pour immediately into pie shell.

Bake pie in lower third of oven on a cookie sheet or pie skirt (filling may boil over), until top is golden and looks dry but filling still trembles, about 45 minutes. Cool on a rack and chill before slicing (filling will sink and set up as it cools).

NUTRIENT ANALYSIS PER SERVING:
Calories (kcal) 213.60

Protein (g) 2.52	Calories from Protein 9.84	% Calories from Protein 4.61
Carbohydrates (g) 39.53	Calories from Carbohydrates 154.61	% Calories from Carbohydrates 72.38
Fat (g) 5.59	Calories from Fat 49.16	% Calories from Fat 23.01
Saturated Fat (g) 0.50	Total Dietary Fiber (g) 0.47	Sodium (mg) 159.65

SWEET CHERRY ALMOND CAKE

∞

*T*his is probably the cake I bake the most. It's fast, easy, low fat, packed with soluble fiber, and has the added goodness of fresh fruit and almonds. It's even low in sugar for a dessert. Most importantly, it's absolutely delicious. If cherries aren't in season, try plums or apricots. I make this cake year 'round with any fruit in season, and I eat it for breakfast as well as dessert.

MAKES 14-16 SERVINGS

¾ cup almonds, finely ground
¾ cup packed brown sugar
⅓ cup plus 3 tablespoons all-purpose unbleached white flour
6 large organic egg whites
¼ teaspoon salt
¼ cup canola oil
1½ teaspoons vanilla
1½ teaspoons almond extract
2 cups cooked cherries (or thinly sliced fresh plums or fresh apricots)
½ teaspoon granulated sugar

Preheat oven to 375°F. Spray a 10" non-stick springform pan with cooking oil and set aside. In a medium bowl whisk together almonds, brown sugar, and flour until well combined. In a large bowl beat egg whites with salt until they just hold stiff peaks and fold in nut mixture gently but thoroughly. Fold in oil, vanilla, and almond extract, and spread batter in prepared pan.

Arrange cherries evenly over batter and sprinkle with granulated sugar. Bake cake for 25–30 minutes or until a tester comes out clean. Cool on rack.

NUTRIENT ANALYSIS PER SERVING:
Calories (kcal) 125.57

Protein (g) 3.18	Calories from Protein 12.24	% Calories from Protein 9.75
Carbohydrates (g) 13.93	Calories from Carbohydrates 53.59	% Calories from Carbohydrates 42.67
Fat (g) 6.90	Calories from Fat 59.74	% Calories from Fat 47.58
Saturated Fat (g) 0.59	Total Dietary Fiber (g) 1.62	Sodium (mg) 60.60

CINNAMON WALNUT TART WITH CRANBERRY RUM SAUCE

∞

This is yet another one of my grandmother's wonderful traditional recipes that required very minor IBS modifications. She served it to company and at Christmas dinner. It is definitely special enough to warrant such a festive occasion. The tart is a rich, gooey, cinnamon-y treat and the Cranberry Rum sauce provides a beautiful jewel-colored note of tart contrast (if cranberries are out of season Raspberry Sauce (page 251) makes a heavenly substitute).

MAKES 10 SERVINGS

CRUST:

8 graham crackers, finely crushed
1 tablespoon canola oil

Preheat oven to 325°F. Lightly spray 9" heavy pie plate with cooking oil. Mix all crust ingredients together thoroughly and press firmly into pan. Bake 4–5 mins. Cool on rack.

FILLING:

1 cup firmly packed brown sugar
4 organic egg whites
½ cup all-purpose unbleached white flour
½ teaspoon baking powder
2 cups finely ground walnuts
½ teaspoon cinnamon

Raise oven temperature to 350°F. In medium bowl, with electric mixer beat sugar and egg whites until creamy. Sift in flour and baking powder, beat briefly, then add nuts and cinnamon. Beat well and pour into cooled crust. Bake 25–35 minutes. Cool on rack before slicing. Serve with Cranberry Rum Sauce or Raspberry Sauce (page 251).

CRANBERRY RUM SAUCE:

1 cup brown sugar
¾ cup water
12 oz. package fresh or frozen cranberries
4 tablespoons spiced rum
½ teaspoon orange oil or orange extract, if desired

Combine water and sugar in medium saucepan. Bring to a boil over medium heat, add cranberries and return to boil. Cook for 10 minutes, or until cranberries pop and mixture thickens, stirring occasionally. Remove from heat and pour mixture through a sieve, pushing hard on solids. Discard solids and stir rum into sauce (and extract). Cool to room temperature before serving.

NUTRIENT ANALYSIS PER SERVING WITHOUT SAUCE:
Calories (kcal) 297.10

Protein (g) 5.87	Calories from Protein 22.49	% Calories from Protein 7.57
Carbohydrates (g) 33.65	Calories from Carbohydrates 129.02	% Calories from Carbohydrates 43.43
Fat (g) 16.88	Calories from Fat 145.58	% Calories from Fat 49.00
Saturated Fat (g) 1.53	Total Dietary Fiber (g) 1.48	Sodium (mg) 82.90

SPICED RUM STRAWBERRY ANGEL FOOD SHORTCAKES

∞

*S*trawberry shortcake is everybody's favorite summertime dessert, but traditional shortcake biscuits are very high in fat. This angel food cake version is a perfectly safe alternative, and is light, sweet, and bursting with berry richness. If you don't have the time to make a cake from scratch, feel free to use a mix.

MAKES 16 SERVINGS

CAKE:*

1 cup cake flour (not self-rising), sifted before measuring
1½ cups granulated sugar
1¾ cups organic egg whites (from about 12–13 large eggs)
1 teaspoon cream of tartar
Dash salt

Preheat oven to 350°F. Sift pre-sifted flour with ¾ cup sugar. Set aside. In a large bowl, beat egg whites with an electric mixer at low speed until frothy and add cream of tartar and salt. Beat whites at high speed until they just form soft peaks. Slowly sift in remaining ¾ cup sugar and beat at high speed, until mixture forms stiff peaks. Gently fold in flour/sugar mixture by hand with rubber spatula in 4 batches until just combined.

Carefully pour batter into an ungreased 10" tube pan with removable bottom, and bake for 35–40 minutes until golden and sides pull away from edges of pan. Immediately invert pan over the neck of a bottle and cool completely. Run a thin knife around edges of cake and remove side of pan. Run the knife under the bottom of the cake and around the center tube and invert cake onto a plate.

Slice the cake and top each piece with a spoonful of the Strawberries in Spiced Rum Syrup.

STRAWBERRIES IN SPICED RUM SYRUP:

1 quart strawberries, hulled and sliced
1 cup granulated sugar
½ cup spiced rum
Zest from one orange

Mix all ingredients except berries in microwave-safe bowl until sugar dissolves. Microwave on high for 3–5 minutes, until mixture boils and slightly reduces. Add strawberries. Let sit at least one hour.

If strawberries are unavailable mangoes make a delicious substitution.

*Please note that angel food cakes, while easy to make, must be made very carefully. Follow the directions precisely, sift as directed, and do not be in a hurry when beating the eggs or adding the sugar. It is also crucial that your electric beaters, bowl, and baking pan be completely grease-free. The tiniest speck of oil, including any wayward flecks of egg yolk, will prevent the whites from whipping properly and the cake from rising.

NUTRIENT ANALYSIS PER SERVING:
Calories (kcal) 192.59

Protein (g) 3.88	Calories from Protein 16.54	% Calories from Protein 8.59
Carbohydrates (g) 40.70	Calories from Carbohydrates 173.73	% Calories from Carbohydrates 90.21
Fat (g) 0.24	Calories from Fat 2.32	% Calories from Fat 1.21
Saturated Fat (g) 0.02	Total Dietary Fiber (g) 1.24	Sodium (mg) 44.67

CLOUD NINE LEMON ANGEL FOOD CAKE WITH CITRUS SYRUP

∞

This is a wonderful dessert that is a lovely light finish to a summer meal. Angel food cakes are the perfect sweet treat for IBS, so indulge without worry.

MAKES 16 SERVINGS

CAKE:*

1 cup cake flour (not self-rising), sifted before measuring
1½ cups granulated sugar
1¾ cups organic egg whites (from about 12–13 large eggs)
1 teaspoon cream of tartar
Dash salt
3 tablespoons freshly grated lemon zest (from about 4 lemons)

Preheat oven to 350°F. Sift pre-sifted flour with ¾ cup sugar. Set aside. In a large bowl, beat egg whites with an electric mixer at low speed until frothy and add cream of tartar and salt. Beat whites at high speed until they just form soft peaks. Slowly sift in remaining ¾ cup sugar and lemon zest, and beat at high speed until mixture forms stiff peaks. Gently fold in flour/sugar mixture by hand with rubber spatula in 4 batches until just combined.

Carefully pour batter into an ungreased 10" tube pan with removable bottom, and bake for 35–40 minutes until golden and sides pull away from edges of pan. Immediately invert pan over the neck of a bottle and cool completely. Run a thin knife around edges of cake and remove side of pan. Run the knife under the bottom of the cake and around the center tube and invert cake onto a plate.

Slice the cake and top each piece with a spoonful of the Citrus Syrup.

CITRUS SYRUP:

¾ cup granulated sugar
½ cup fresh lemon juice
½ cup fresh orange juice

In a small saucepan combine all ingredients and cook over medium heat until sugar dissolves and syrup is slightly thickened, about 5 minutes.

*Please note that angel food cakes, while easy to make, must be made very carefully. Follow the directions precisely, sift as directed, and do not be in a hurry when beating the eggs or adding the sugar. It is also crucial that your electric beaters, bowl, and baking pan be completely grease-free. The tiniest speck of oil, including any wayward flecks of egg yolk, will prevent the whites from whipping properly and the cake from rising.

NUTRIENT ANALYSIS PER SERVING:
Calories (kcal) 156.45

Protein (g) 3.69	Calories from Protein 14.49	% Calories from Protein 9.26
Carbohydrates (g) 35.91	Calories from Carbohydrates 141.15	% Calories from Carbohydrates 90.22
Fat (g) 0.09	Calories from Fat 0.81	% Calories from Fat 0.52
Saturated Fat (g) 0.01	Total Dietary Fiber (g) 0.26	Sodium (mg) 44.28

MENUS
AT-A-GLANCE

∞

I'VE TRIED TO structure these suggested daily meal plans for maximum convenience. Many of the items listed can be prepared well in advance and will keep for many days in the fridge to be used as needed throughout the week. Dinner for one night is typically served as lunch the next day, and homemade bread serves as snacks, breakfasts, and desserts.

Please don't feel obligated to follow these menus precisely. I've tried to design very generous daily suggestions, both in terms of variety and quantity. You can easily reduce the scale and make changes or substitutions. The important thing is to follow the basic formula of having soluble fiber as the basis for each meal or snack, the first thing you always eat, and the item you eat in the greatest quantity.

Day 1

BREAKFAST   Blueberry Brown Sugar Scottish Oatmeal.

SNACK   Home dried bananas.* Glass of soy milk.

LUNCH   Baguette sandwich with rosemary fig chutney and shaved smoked chicken breast.* Crunchy pizza party snack mix.* Four stalks of steamed fresh asparagus, sprinkled with fresh lemon juice and garlic salt. Small pear. Mint tea.

SNACK   Slice of sweet cinnamon zucchini bread.*

DINNER   Baked corn chips. Sizzling shrimp fajitas with Baja orange marinade,* smoky black bean dip,* fresh Tex-Mex guacamole,* and sweet mango and roasted tomato salsa.* Mexican cinnamon lime horchata.*

Day 2

BREAKFAST   Sweet cinnamon zucchini bread.* Glass of Mexican cinnamon lime horchata.*

SNACK   Handful of home dried bananas.* Mint tea

LUNCH   Baked corn chips with smoky black bean dip,* fresh Tex-Mex guacamole,* and sweet mango roasted tomato salsa.* Chocolate silk pudding.*

SNACK   Handful of fat-free crackers or Crunchy pizza party snack mix.*

DINNER   French bread. Linguine with creamy wild mushroom, spinach, and sherry sauce.* Sweet mango and roasted tomato salsa. Tart cranberry, lime, and honey refresher.* Will's dreamy lemon rice pudding.*

Day 3

BREAKFAST   *Will's dreamy lemon rice pudding.* Mint tea.

SNACK   *Sweet cinnamon zucchini bread.**

LUNCH   *French bread. Linguine with creamy wild mushroom, spinach, and sherry sauce.* Small diced mango or 4 small strawberries. Mint tea.*

SNACK   *Chocolate silk pudding.**

DINNER   *Italian crostini with honey-tomato sauce and garlic saffron prawns.* Small handful of steamed fresh green beans, sprinkled with fresh lemon juice and garlic salt. Small banana.*

Day 4

BREAKFAST   *Pumpkin apple spice bread.* Glass of soy milk.*

SNACK   *Home dried bananas.* Mint tea.*

LUNCH   *Italian crostini with honey-tomato sauce and garlic saffron prawns .* Small portion of steamed fresh zucchini. Slice of better than cheesecake with summer fruit topping.**

SNACK   *Handful of pretzels.*

DINNER   *Japanese soba noodles with benito dipping sauce.* Steamed sweet potatoes with Japanese miso dressing.* Handful of Japanese-style steamed fresh soy beans.* Small pear. Green tea with honey.**

Day 5

BREAKFAST Pumpkin apple spice bread.* Glass of soy or rice milk.

SNACK Slice of better than cheesecake.* Mint tea.

LUNCH Japanese soba noodles with benito dipping sauce,* steamed sweet potatoes with Japanese miso dressing.,* Japanese-style steamed fresh soy beans.* Asian sweet pickled cucumbers.* Small slice of melon or banana.

SNACK Crunchy pizza party snack mix.*

DINNER French bread. Maple-glazed salmon with nuttywheat berries.* Small portion of steamed fresh peeled zucchini with fresh lemon juice and garlic salt. Slice of better than cheesecake.* Mint tea.

Day 6

BREAKFAST Banana-banana bread French toast.* Hearty Mexican omelette.* Mint tea.

SNACK Slice of pumpkin apple spice bread.* Glass of soy milk.

LUNCH French bread. Maple-glazed salmon with nuttywheat berries.* Handful of steamed fresh broccoli with fresh lemon juice and garlic salt. Slice of better than cheesecake.*

SNACK Home dried bananas.*

DINNER Baked potato chips. Louisiana barbecued catfish sandwiches with sweet and sour wilted cabbage slaw.* Candied sweet potatoes.* Pucker up, Buttercup Lemon sorbet.*

Day 7

BREAKFAST   Brown sugar banana bread. Glass of soy or rice milk.

SNACK   Handful of pretzels. Mint tea.

LUNCH   Baked potato chips. Louisiana barbecued catfish sandwiches with sweet and sour wilted cabbage slaw.* Candied sweet potatoes.* Small portion baked beans. Pucker up, Buttercup Lemon sorbet.*

SNACK   Crunchy pizza party snack mix.* Mint tea.

DINNER   Fresh Jasmine rice. Orange-glazed chicken breast with onions, mushrooms, and carrots.* Small portion steamed fresh broccoli. Spiced rum strawberry angle food shortcakes..

*Recipes included

DIRECTORY OF RESOURCES

∞

𝓜ost, if not all, recipe ingredients should be easily available through your local supermarkets and health and specialty food stores, but if not these stores can supply them.

ADRIANA'S CARAVAN
(Asian ingredients)
1-800-316-0820

CHILE TODAY, HOT TAMALE
(dried chipotle and other peppers)
www.chiletoday.com
1-800-HOT-PEPPER

GREAT AMERICAN SPICE COMPANY
(mesquite smoke powder)
www.americanspice.com

HELP FOR IBS
(Acacia Tummy Fiber, Tummy Tamers enteric coated peppermint capsules and fennel oil capsules, Peppermint and Fennel Tummy teas)
1-866-640-4942
www.HelpForIBS.com

IBS HYPNOTHERAPY CDs
www.HelpForIBS.com
Phone: 1-866-640-4942
Mail: Michael Mahoney, Clinical Hypnotherapist
Guardian Medical Centre
Guardian St. Warrington Cheshire
WA5 1UD
England
Cost: $88 U.S.

KALUSTYAN'S
(Indian and Middle Eastern ingredients)
www.kalustyans.com
1-212-685-3451

KITCHEN MARKET
(Mexican ingredients)
1-888-468-4433

MO HOTTA MO BETTA
(dried chipotle and other peppers)
www.mohotta.com
1-800-462-3220

UWAJIMAYA'S
(Asian ingredients)
1-800-889-1928

WHOLE FOODS
(soy/rice milk, soy substitutes for dairy products, general health food store items)
www.wholefoods.com
1-888-945-3637

RECOMMENDED READING
∞

Michael D. Gershon. *The Second Brain: A Groundbreaking New Understanding of Nervous Disorders of the Stomach and Intestine*, Harper Perennial Library, 1999.

John Robbins. *Diet for a New America: How Your Food Choices Affect Your Health, Happiness and the Future of Life on Earth*, H.J. Kramer, 1998.

ABOUT THE AUTHOR
∞

HEATHER VAN VOROUS is a food writer specializing in recipes for people with bowel disorders and lactose intolerance. She has suffered from IBS since age nine, although she went undiagnosed until age fifteen. Over the course of twenty years she gradually learned how to control her IBS symptoms through dietary modifications, while at the same time pursuing her interest in gourmet cooking and ethnic foods. She has combined these two areas of expertise in this book. Heather received a BA in 1992 from the University of Puget Sound, Tacoma, Washington, and an MA in 1996 from the University of Massachusetts, Amherst.

INDEX